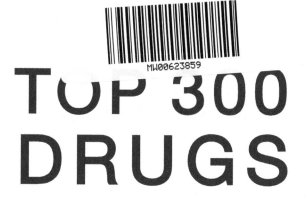

TOP 300
DRUGS
Pocket Reference Guide

ACYCLOVIR

Brand Names
- Zovirax, Sitavig, Avaclyr

Pharmacologic Class
- Antiviral

Mechanism of Action
- Acyclovir is converted to the active triphosphate form, which interferes with viral DNA polymerase and inhibits viral DNA replication.

Dosage Forms
- Oral (tablet, buccal tablet, capsule, suspension), topical (ointment, cream), intravenous (solution)

Common Uses
- Treatment of genital herpes, herpes zoster (shingles), and varicella zoster (chickenpox)

Quick Facts
- Reduce dosage in renal impairment (CrCl < 25 mL/min/1.73 m^2).
- Infuse IV form over at least 1 hour and avoid IV push, IM, or SubQ injection.
- Wear rubber gloves when applying ointment or cream to prevent virus transmission to other parts of the body.
- Drink plenty of fluids when using oral form to prevent renal toxicity.
- Side effects: diarrhea, nausea, vomiting, headache

ADALIMUMAB

Brand Name
- Humira

Pharmacologic Class
- TNFα inhibitor

Mechanism of Action
- Binds to TNFα and prevents its interaction with cell surface TNF receptors, thereby inhibiting cytokine-driven inflammatory processes.

Dosage Form
- Subcutaneous (solution)

Common Uses
- Treatment of rheumatoid arthritis, psoriatic arthritis, Chron's disease, and ulcerative colitis

Quick Facts
- Black Box Warning – Patients are at an increased risk of serious infections leading to hospitalization or death, including tuberculosis (TB), bacterial sepsis, invasive fungal infections, and infections due to other opportunistic pathogens. Lymphoma and other malignancies have been reported.
- Avoid live vaccines during therapy.
- All patients should be screened for TB before and during therapy.
- Side effects: injection site pain or reaction, rash, headache, upper respiratory tract infection, sinusitis

ALBUTEROL

Brand Names
- ProAir, Ventolin, Proventil

Pharmacologic Class
- Beta$_2$-agonist

Mechanism of Action
- Relaxes bronchial smooth muscle by binding to beta$_2$-adrenergic receptors.

Dosage Forms
- Inhalation (powder, solution, suspension), oral (tablet, syrup)

Common Uses
- Treatment of asthma, exercise-induced asthma, COPD, and bronchospasm

Quick Facts
- HFA inhalers should be shaken well before each use. Prime prior to first use and when inhaler has not been used for more than 2 weeks by spraying into air 3 to 4 times.
- Mouthpiece of HFA inhalers should be cleaned at least once per week by removing the canister and running under warm water, then air-drying completely.
- Side effects: palpitations, tremors, dizziness, cough, nervousness

ALBUTEROL-IPRATROPIUM

Brand Names
- Combivent Respimat, DuoNeb

Pharmacologic Class
- Combination $beta_2$-agonist and anticholinergic

Mechanism of Action
- Albuterol relaxes bronchial smooth muscle by binding to $beta_2$-adrenergic receptors, and ipratropium blocks the action of acetylcholine at parasympathetic sites in bronchial smooth muscle causing bronchodilation.

Dosage Forms
- Inhalation (solution, aerosol powder, spray)

Common Use
- Treatment of COPD

Quick Facts
- Avoid spraying in or near eyes as this may cause eye pain, temporary blurring of vision, visual halos, mydriasis, or new onset or worsening of narrow-angle glaucoma.
- Use with caution in patients with narrow-angle glaucoma, BPH, or bladder neck obstruction.
- Soft-mist inhaler should be primed prior to first use or if not used in more than 21 days.
- Clean mouthpiece of soft-mist inhaler at least once per week with a damp cloth or tissue.
- Side effects: dry mouth, upper respiratory tract infection, sinusitis

ALENDRONATE

Brand Names
- Fosamax, Binosto

Pharmacologic Class
- Bisphosphonate

Mechanism of Action
- Inhibits osteoclast-mediated bone resorption.

Dosage Forms
- Oral (tablet, effervescent tablet, solution)

Common Uses
- Treatment and prevention of osteoporosis; treatment of Paget's disease

Quick Facts
- Medication should be taken in the morning at least 30 minutes before the first food, beverage, and other medications of the day. Patient should stay upright for at least 30 minutes and until after eating to prevent esophageal irritation.
- Oral tablet should be taken with 6 to 8 oz. of plain water, and oral solution should be followed with at least 2 oz. of plain water.
- Side effects: abdominal pain, acid regurgitation, constipation, diarrhea, and esophagitis
- Less common side effects: osteonecrosis of the jaw, atypical femur fracture

ALLOPURINOL

Brand Names
- Zyloprim, Aloprim

Pharmacologic Class
- Xanthine oxidase inhibitor

Mechanism of Action
- Decreases the production of uric acid by inhibiting the action of xanthine oxidase.

Dosage Forms
- Oral (tablet), intravenous (powder for solution)

Common Uses
- Treatment of gout; prevention of tumor lysis syndrome and recurrent nephrolithiasis

Quick Facts
- Reduce dosage in renal impairment (CrCl < 20 mL/min).
- Take medication after meals to reduce gastric irritation.
- Patients should be counseled to immediately report a skin rash as it can develop into Stevens-Johnson syndrome or toxic epidermal necrolysis.
- Medication may take several weeks to have an effect.
- Side effects: diarrhea, nausea, precipitation of acute gout attacks

ALPRAZOLAM

Brand Name
- Xanax

Pharmacologic Class
- Benzodiazepine

Mechanism of Action
- Causes CNS depression by potentiating the effects of GABA (an inhibitory neurotransmitter).

Dosage Forms
- Oral (tablet, disintegrating tablet, solution)

Common Uses
- Treatment of anxiety disorders and panic disorder

Quick Facts
- DEA Schedule IV
- Black Box Warning – Concomitant use with opioids increases risk of sedation, respiratory depression, coma, or death.
- Avoid abrupt discontinuation to prevent withdrawal symptoms.
- Avoid alcohol, grapefruit, and grapefruit juice.
- Dose adjustment recommended in advanced liver disease.
- Side effects: drowsiness, dizziness, ataxia, lightheadedness

AMIODARONE

Brand Names
- Cordarone, Pacerone

Pharmacologic Class
- Antiarrhythmic (Class III)

Mechanism of Action
- Primarily blocks potassium channels, increasing the duration of the action potential and refractory period in myocardial tissue. Also interferes with the functioning of beta-adrenergic receptors, sodium channels, and calcium channels.

Dosage Forms
- Oral (tablet), intravenous (solution)

Common Uses
- Treatment and prevention of ventricular arrhythmia

Quick Facts
- Black Box Warning – Risk of pulmonary toxicity, hepatotoxicity, and worsened arrhythmia. Treatment should be initiated in a clinical setting.
- Monitor pulmonary function, thyroid function, and liver function. Perform baseline and regular ophthalmic exams.
- Avoid St. John's wort and grapefruit juice.
- Side effects: hypotension, heart block, pulmonary fibrosis, sinus bradycardia, skin discoloration, hypothyroidism, hyperthyroidism, corneal deposits, optic neuropathy

AMITRIPTYLINE

Brand Name
- Elavil

Pharmacologic Class
- Tricyclic antidepressant

Mechanism of Action
- Increases the synaptic concentration of serotonin and norepinephrine in the CNS by inhibiting their reuptake at presynaptic nerve terminals.

Dosage Form
- Oral (tablet)

Common Uses
- Treatment of depression and neuropathic pain; migraine prevention

Quick Facts
- Black Box Warning – Increased risk of suicidal thoughts and behavior, especially in children, adolescents, and young adults.
- Can prolong the QT interval.
- Do not abruptly discontinue medication.
- Symptomatic improvement may take several weeks.
- Use is contraindicated during or within 14 days of MAOI administration.
- Side effects: dry mouth, blurred vision, urinary retention, constipation, weight gain, drowsiness

AMLODIPINE

Brand Names
- Norvasc, Katerzia

Pharmacologic Class
- Calcium channel blocker

Mechanism of Action
- Dihydropyridine CCB that blocks the transmembrane influx of calcium ions into vascular smooth muscle and cardiac muscle which results in increased peripheral arterial vasodilation and decreased peripheral vascular resistance.

Dosage Forms
- Oral (tablet, suspension)

Common Uses
- Treatment of chronic stable angina and variant angina, hypertension

Quick Facts
- May worsen angina and increase the risk of MI after starting or increasing dose.
- Risk of peripheral edema can be minimized if medication is administered at bedtime and lower doses are used (2.5 or 5 mg/day).
- Side effects: peripheral edema, fatigue, reflex tachycardia, headache, flushing

AMLODIPINE-BENAZEPRIL

Brand Name
- Lotrel

Pharmacologic Class
- Combination calcium channel blocker and ACE inhibitor

Mechanism of Action
- Amlodipine is a dihydropyridine CCB that blocks the transmembrane influx of calcium ions into vascular smooth muscle and cardiac muscle which results in increased peripheral arterial vasodilation and decreased peripheral vascular resistance. Benazepril inhibits the angiotensin converting enzyme (ACE), which prevents the conversion of angiotensin I to angiotensin II, a potent vasoconstrictor.

Dosage Form
- Oral (capsule)

Common Use
- Treatment of hypertension

Quick Facts
- Black Box Warning – Discontinue use as soon as possible if pregnancy is detected.
- Contraindicated in patients with history of angioedema, concomitant use with aliskiren in diabetic patients, concomitant use with neprilysin inhibitor, or within 36 hours of switching to or from a neprilysin inhibitor.
- Use caution in patients with impaired renal function.
- Patients should avoid potassium supplements or salt substitutes containing potassium without first consulting healthcare provider.
- Side effects: cough, headache, edema, angioedema

AMOXICILLIN

Brand Names
- Amoxil, Trimox, Moxatag

Pharmacologic Class
- Penicillin antibiotic

Mechanism of Action
- Inhibits bacterial cell wall synthesis by binding to one or more of the penicillin-binding proteins, which inhibits the final transpeptidation step of peptidoglycan synthesis in bacterial cell walls.

Dosage Forms
- Oral (tablet, capsule, powder for suspension, chewable tablet)

Common Uses
- Treatment of ear, nose, and throat infections (pharyngitis/tonsillitis, otitis media), genitourinary tract infections, *H. pylori* eradication, lower respiratory tract infections, skin and soft tissue infections, and sinusitis

Quick Facts
- Keep suspension refrigerated and discard after 14 days.
- Take at even intervals, preferably around the clock.
- Side effects: diarrhea, nausea, vomiting, rash

AMOXICILLIN-CLAVULANATE

Brand Name
- Augmentin

Pharmacologic Class
- Penicillin antibiotic

Mechanism of Action
- Amoxicillin inhibits bacterial cell wall synthesis by binding to one or more of the penicillin-binding proteins, which inhibits the final transpeptidation step of peptidoglycan synthesis in bacterial cell walls. Clavulanate inactivates beta-lactamase enzymes, which protects amoxicillin from degradation and increases its spectrum of activity.

Dosage Forms
- Oral (tablet, powder for suspension, chewable tablet)

Common Uses
- Treatment of acute otitis media, community-acquired pneumonia, sinusitis, skin and skin structure infections, and UTIs

Quick Facts
- Keep suspension refrigerated and discard after 10 days.
- Take at the start of a meal to increase absorption and decrease GI upset.
- Side effects: diarrhea, nausea, vomiting, rash

AMPHETAMINE-DEXTROAMPHETAMINE

Brand Names
- Adderall, Mydayis

Pharmacologic Class
- CNS stimulant

Mechanism of Action
- Blocks the reuptake of norepinephrine and dopamine in presynaptic nerve endings and increases their release into the extraneuronal space.

Dosage Forms
- Oral (tablet, capsule)

Common Uses
- Treatment of ADHD and narcolepsy

Quick Facts
- DEA Schedule II
- Black Box Warning – High potential for abuse, and administration for prolonged periods of time may lead to dependence. Misuse may cause sudden death and serious cardiovascular adverse reactions.
- Use is contraindicated during or within 14 days of MAOI administration, including linezolid or methylene blue.
- Gradually increase dosing and avoid abrupt discontinuation to prevent withdrawal symptoms.
- Use with caution in patients with a history of seizures.
- Side effects: loss of appetite, weight loss, restlessness, nervousness, nausea, diarrhea

ANASTROZOLE

Brand Name
- Arimidex

Pharmacologic Class
- Aromatase inhibitor

Mechanism of Action
- Non-steroidal aromatase inhibitor that blocks the conversion of androgens to estrogens in peripheral tissues.

Dosage Form
- Oral (tablet)

Common Use
- Treatment of breast cancer in postmenopausal women

Quick Facts
- Can decrease bone mineral density. (Monitor at baseline and every 1 to 2 years with DEXA scan.)
- Consider monitoring total cholesterol and LDL during therapy.
- Use is not recommended in premenopausal women.
- Side effects: hot flashes, fatigue, nausea, vomiting, rash

APIXABAN

Brand Name
- Eliquis

Pharmacologic Class
- Factor Xa inhibitor

Mechanism of Action
- Reversible and selective active site inhibitor of free and clot-bound factor Xa, resulting in decreased thrombin generation and thrombus formation.

Dosage Form
- Oral (tablet)

Common Uses
- Treatment and prophylaxis of DVT or PE; used to reduce the risk of stroke and systemic embolism in patients with nonvalvular atrial fibrillation (AF); prophylaxis of DVT in patients who have undergone hip or knee replacement surgery

Quick Facts
- Black Box Warnings – Premature discontinuation increases the risk of thrombotic events. To reduce risk consider coverage with another anticoagulant if apixaban is discontinued for a reason other than pathological bleeding or completion of therapy. Patients undergoing neuroaxial anesthesia or spinal puncture have an increased risk of epidural or spinal hematomas which could result in permanent paralysis.
- Dosage adjustment required in patients with renal impairment and nonvalvular atrial fibrillation (2.5 mg twice daily in patients with at least two of the following characteristics: age ≥ 80 years, body weight ≤ 60 kg, or serum creatinine ≥ 1.5 mg/dL).
- Side effects: hemorrhage, bruising, syncope, anemia

ARIPIPRAZOLE

Brand Name
- Abilify

Pharmacologic Class
- Antipsychotic

Mechanism of Action
- May exert its effects through partial agonist activity at the dopamine D_2 and serotonin $5\text{-}HT_{1A}$ receptors, and antagonist activity at serotonin $5\text{-}HT_{2A}$ receptors.

Dosage Forms
- Oral (tablet, disintegrating tablet, solution), intramuscular (powder for suspension)

Common Uses
- Treatment of bipolar disorder, schizophrenia, major depressive disorder, Tourette's syndrome, and irritability associated with autistic disorder

Quick Facts
- Black Box Warnings – Elderly patients with dementia-related psychosis treated with antipsychotic drugs are at an increased risk of death. There is an increased risk of suicidal thoughts and behavior in children, adolescents, and young adults.
- May prolong the QT interval.
- Patients should be counseled to report signs of extrapyramidal symptoms, tardive dyskinesia (restlessness, tremor, stiffness, etc.), or neuroleptic malignant syndrome (sweating, fever, muscle rigidity).
- Monitor for hyperglycemia, dyslipidemia, and weight gain.
- Side effects: anxiety, insomnia, nausea, headache

ASPIRIN-DIPYRIDAMOLE

Brand Name
- Aggrenox

Pharmacologic Class
- Antiplatelet

Mechanism of Action
- Aspirin inhibits platelet aggregation by irreversibly inhibiting platelet cyclooxygenase, which prevents the production of thromboxane A_2. Dipyridamole inhibits the reuptake of adenosine into platelets, endothelial cells, and erythrocytes, which increases levels of cAMP and further inhibits platelet aggregation.

Dosage Form
- Oral (capsule)

Common Use
- For secondary stroke prevention in patients who have had a transient ischemic attack (TIA) or ischemic stroke due to thrombosis

Quick Facts
- Patients should avoid additional aspirin or aspirin-containing products without consulting their prescriber.
- Patients who consume 3 or more alcoholic drinks daily should be counseled about bleeding risks with aspirin.
- Side effects: headache, dyspepsia, abdominal pain, nausea, diarrhea, bleeding

ATENOLOL

Brand Name
- Tenormin

Pharmacologic Class
- Beta$_1$-selective blocker

Mechanism of Action
- Binds to the beta$_1$-adrenergic receptors found in vascular smooth muscle and the heart, blocking the positive inotropic and chronotropic actions of endogenous catecholamines such as isoproterenol, norepinephrine, and epinephrine.

Dosage Forms
- Oral (tablet, powder for solution)

Common Uses
- Treatment of hypertension, acute MI, and angina pectoris (chronic)

Quick Facts
- Black Box Warning – Abrupt cessation may precipitate angina, MI, arrhythmias, or rebound hypertension.
- Contraindicated in patients with AV block, bradycardia, cardiogenic shock, and overt heart failure.
- Medication can mask symptoms of hypoglycemia in diabetics.
- Side effects: bradycardia, hypotension, dizziness, fatigue

ATENOLOL-CHLORTHALIDONE

Brand Name
- Tenoretic

Pharmacologic Class
- Combination $beta_1$-selective blocker and thiazide diuretic

Mechanism of Action
- Atenolol binds to the $beta_1$-adrenergic receptors found in vascular smooth muscle and the heart, blocking the positive inotropic and chronotropic actions of endogenous catecholamines such as isoproterenol, norepinephrine, and epinephrine. Chlorthalidone inhibits sodium and chloride reabsorption in the renal distal convoluted tubule.

Dosage Form
- Oral (tablet)

Common Use
- Treatment of hypertension

Quick Facts
- Contraindicated in patients with AV block, bradycardia, cardiogenic shock, overt heart failure, anuria, and hypersensitivity to sulfonamides.
- Administer in the morning because of increased diuresis.
- Avoid abrupt discontinuation of medication to prevent rebound hypertension.
- Side effects: orthostatic hypotension, dizziness, fatigue, bradycardia, dyspnea

ATOMOXETINE

Brand Name
- Strattera

Pharmacologic Class
- Norepinephrine reuptake inhibitor

Mechanism of Action
- Selective inhibitor of the norepinephrine transporter, which prevents cellular reuptake of norepinephrine throughout the brain.

Dosage Form
- Oral (capsule)

Common Use
- Treatment of ADHD

Quick Facts
- Black Box Warning – Increased risk of suicidal ideation in children and adolescents.
- Use is contraindicated during or within 14 days of MAOI administration, or in patients with narrow-angle glaucoma or pheochromocytoma.
- Patients should be advised to report symptoms of liver injury or cardiovascular problems, which include chest pain, palpitations, and dyspnea.
- Do not crush, chew, or open capsule.
- Side effects: dry mouth, fatigue, mood swings, appetite suppression, dysmenorrhea

ATORVASTATIN

Brand Name
- Lipitor

Pharmacologic Class
- HMG-CoA reductase inhibitor

Mechanism of Action
- Inhibits HMG-CoA reductase, preventing the conversion of HMG-CoA to mevalonate (the rate-limiting step in cholesterol synthesis).

Dosage Form
- Oral (tablet)

Common Use
- Treatment of hyperlipidemia

Quick Facts
- Contraindicated in active liver disease and in pregnancy and lactation.
- CYP3A4 inhibitors can increase plasma concentration.
- Monitor LFTs at baseline and periodically thereafter.
- Limit alcohol intake and avoid grapefruit and grapefruit juice.
- Can be taken at any time of day.
- Side effects: diarrhea, arthralgia, myalgia, increased liver enzymes, UTIs, nasopharyngitis

AZATHIOPRINE

Brand Names
- Azasan, Imuran

Pharmacologic Class
- Immunosuppressant

Mechanism of Action
- Inhibits purine synthesis, causing less DNA and RNA to be produced for the synthesis of white blood cells.

Dosage Forms
- Oral (tablet), intravenous (powder for solution)

Common Uses
- Treatment of rheumatoid arthritis; prevention of organ rejection in renal transplants

Quick Facts
- Black Box Warning – Increases risk of malignancy. Reports include post-transplant lymphoma and hepatosplenic T-cell lymphoma (HSTCL) in patients with inflammatory bowel disease.
- Taking medication with meals and/or in divided doses may decrease adverse GI events.
- Monitor CBC and LFTs during therapy.
- Side effects: diarrhea, nausea, vomiting, hepatotoxicity, increased susceptibility to infections, bone marrow suppression

AZELASTINE (nasal)

Brand Names
- Astelin, Astepro

Pharmacologic Class
- H_1 antagonist

Mechanism of Action
- Histamine H_1 receptor antagonist that inhibits the release of histamine from cells involved in the allergic response.

Dosage Form
- Nasal (solution)

Common Uses
- Treatment of perennial and seasonal allergic rhinitis, vasomotor rhinitis

Quick Facts
- Counsel patients to use caution when engaging in activities requiring mental alertness until medication effects are realized, as it may cause somnolence.
- Avoid alcohol and other CNS depressants because of additional reductions in alertness.
- Prime delivery device with 4 sprays of Astelin or 6 sprays of Astepro before initial use and with 2 sprays if not used for 3 or more days.
- Side effects: headache, epistaxis, dysgeusia, fatigue, dizziness

AZITHROMYCIN (systemic)

Brand Names
- Zithromax, Zmax, Z-Pak, Tri-Pak

Pharmacologic Class
- Macrolide antibiotic

Mechanism of Action
- Binds to the 50S subunit of the bacterial ribosome, which inhibits RNA-dependent protein synthesis.

Dosage Forms
- Oral (tablet, powder for suspension), intravenous (powder for solution)

Common Uses
- Treatment of community-acquired pneumonia, acute otitis media, COPD exacerbations, chlamydia, gonorrhea, and skin and soft tissue infections

Quick Facts
- Use with caution in patients with CrCl < 10 mL/min.
- Avoid concomitant use of aluminum or magnesium-containing antacids with tablet and immediate-release suspension.
- Do not refrigerate oral suspension.
- Patients should report symptoms of hepatotoxicity or severe diarrhea.
- Can prolong the QT interval.
- Side effects: diarrhea, nausea, vomiting, abdominal pain

BACLOFEN

Brand Names
- Lioresal, Gablofen, Ozobax

Pharmacologic Class
- Skeletal muscle relaxant

Mechanism of Action
- Believed to work at the spinal level to inhibit transmission of both monosynaptic and polysynaptic reflexes. Baclofen is a structural analog of GABA and binds to the GABA-B receptor, which decreases the release of excitatory neurotransmitters and substance P.

Dosage Forms
- Oral (tablet, solution), intrathecal (solution)

Common Uses
- Treatment of spasticity, muscle spasm not due to rheumatic conditions, myoclonus, and muscle rigidity in multiple sclerosis and spinal cord injury or diseases

Quick Facts
- Avoid abrupt discontinuation to prevent withdrawal symptoms (sedation, somnolence and weakness, psychological symptoms).
- Avoid alcohol and other CNS depressants.
- Side effects: drowsiness, weakness, dizziness, confusion

BECLOMETHASONE
(inhalation)

Brand Name
- Qvar RediHaler

Pharmacologic Class
- Corticosteroid

Mechanism of Action
- Inhibits inflammatory cells (mast cells, eosinophils, basophils, lymphocytes, macrophages, and neutrophils) and release of inflammatory mediators (histamine, eicosanoids, leukotrienes, and cytokines).

Dosage Form
- Inhalation (breath-actuated aerosol)

Common Use
- Treatment of asthma

Quick Facts
- Inhaler device does not require priming or shaking prior to use. Do not use with a spacer or holding chamber. Do not open white cap until ready to use, and if more than one inhalation is needed per dose, close white cap prior to next inhalation.
- Counsel patients to rinse mouth with water, without swallowing, after each use to prevent oral candidiasis.
- Side effects: upper respiratory tract infection, nasopharyngitis, allergic rhinitis, sinusitis, oropharyngeal pain

BENAZEPRIL

Brand Name
- Lotensin

Pharmacologic Class
- ACE inhibitor

Mechanism of Action
- Inhibits the angiotensin converting enzyme (ACE), which prevents the conversion of angiotensin I to angiotensin II, a potent vasoconstrictor.

Dosage Form
- Oral (tablet)

Common Use
- Treatment of hypertension

Quick Facts
- Black Box Warning – Discontinue use as soon as possible if pregnancy is detected.
- Patients should avoid potassium supplements or salt substitutes containing potassium without first consulting healthcare provider.
- Contraindicated in patients with a history of angioedema, concomitant use with aliskiren in diabetic patients, concomitant use with neprilysin inhibitor, or within 36 hours of switching to or from a neprilysin inhibitor.
- Side effects: cough, edema, angioedema, headache, dizziness

BENZONATATE

Brand Name
- Tessalon Perles

Pharmacologic Class
- Antitussive

Mechanism of Action
- Suppresses cough by topical anesthetic action on the stretch receptors located in the respiratory passages, lungs, and pleura.

Dosage Form
- Oral (capsule)

Common Use
- Symptomatic relief of cough

Quick Facts
- Swallow capsule whole, do not chew or dissolve in mouth. (Oropharyngeal anesthesia may occur.)
- Do not use in children < 10 years old.
- Use with caution in patients with a sensitivity to anesthetic agents of the para-aminobenzoic acid class (procaine, tetracaine).
- Side effects: drowsiness, headache, constipation

BENZTROPINE

Brand Name
- Cogentin

Pharmacologic Class
- Anticholinergic

Mechanism of Action
- Inhibits the reuptake and storage of dopamine in CNS cells, and also has anticholinergic and antihistaminic activity.

Dosage Forms
- Oral (tablet), injection solution (IM/IV)

Common Uses
- Treatment of Parkinson's disease and drug-induced extrapyramidal symptoms

Quick Facts
- May take with food or milk to decrease GI upset.
- Medication may produce anhidrosis. Use caution during hot weather and with activities leading to an increase in core temperature or dehydration.
- Medication should not be used in patients with tardive dyskinesia as it can aggravate or unmask symptoms.
- Side effects: dry mouth, constipation, urinary retention, blurred vision

BIMATOPROST

Brand Name
- Lumigan

Pharmacologic Class
- Prostaglandin analog

Mechanism of Action
- Decreases intraocular pressure by increasing the outflow of aqueous humor through the trabecular meshwork and uveoscleral pathway.

Dosage Form
- Ophthalmic (solution)

Common Uses
- Treatment of open-angle glaucoma and ocular hypertension

Quick Facts
- Remove contact lenses before instilling medication and allow at least 15 minutes before reinserting.
- Wait at least 5 minutes before administering other ophthalmic products.
- Blot excess medication to avoid running onto cheek and other skin surfaces, as repeated contact can cause hair growth.
- Side effects: pigment changes to eyelids and eyelashes, increased brown pigmentation of the iris, growth of eyelashes, conjunctival hyperemia, ocular pruritis

BISOPROLOL-HYDROCHLOROTHIAZIDE

Brand Name
- Ziac

Pharmacologic Class
- Combination $beta_1$-selective blocker and thiazide diuretic

Mechanism of Action
- Bisoprolol binds to the $beta_1$-adrenergic receptors found in vascular smooth muscle and the heart, blocking the positive inotropic and chronotropic actions of endogenous catecholamines. Hydrochlorothiazide inhibits sodium and chloride reabsorption in the renal distal convoluted tubule.

Dosage Form
- Oral (tablet)

Common Use
- Treatment of hypertension

Quick Facts
- Administer in the morning because of increased diuresis.
- Contraindicated in patients with AV block, bradycardia, cardiogenic shock, overt heart failure, anuria, and hypersensitivity to sulfonamides.
- Avoid abrupt discontinuation of medication because this can exacerbate angina or induce MI.
- Side effects: fatigue, headache, dizziness

BRIMONIDINE (ophthalmic)

Brand Name
- Alphagan P

Pharmacologic Class
- Alpha$_2$-agonist

Mechanism of Action
- Decreases intraocular pressure by reducing aqueous humor production and increasing uveoscleral outflow.

Dosage Form
- Ophthalmic (solution)

Common Uses
- Treatment of open-angle glaucoma and ocular hypertension

Quick Facts
- Wait at least 5 minutes before administering other ophthalmic products.
- Use with caution with concomitant use of MAOIs due to increased risk of hypotension.
- Tricyclic antidepressants may decrease effectiveness of brimonidine.
- Side effects: allergic conjunctivitis, conjunctival hyperemia, ocular pruritis, hypertension, dry mouth

BUDESONIDE (inhalation)

Brand Name
- Pulmicort

Pharmacologic Class
- Corticosteroid

Mechanism of Action
- Inhibits inflammatory cells (mast cells, eosinophils, basophils, lymphocytes, macrophages, and neutrophils) and release of inflammatory mediators (histamine, eicosanoids, leukotrienes, and cytokines).

Dosage Forms
- Inhalation (suspension, breath-actuated aerosol)

Common Use
- Treatment of asthma

Quick Facts
- Do not shake inhaler device prior to use. Device needs primed prior to first use only. Do not use with a spacer or holding chamber.
- Shake nebulizer suspension well before using.
- Counsel patients to rinse mouth with water, without swallowing, after each use to prevent oral candidiasis, and wash face if using face mask with nebulizer treatment.
- Side effects: oral candidiasis, upper respiratory tract infection, nasopharyngitis, allergic rhinitis, sinusitis

BUDESONIDE-FORMOTEROL

Brand Name
- Symbicort

Pharmacologic Class
- Combination $beta_2$-agonist and corticosteroid

Mechanism of Action
- Budesonide inhibits inflammatory cells (mast cells, eosinophils, basophils, lymphocytes, macrophages, and neutrophils) and release of inflammatory mediators (histamine, eicosanoids, leukotrienes, and cytokines). Formoterol binds to $beta_2$-adrenergic receptors and increases the level of cAMP, which relaxes bronchial smooth muscle.

Dosage Form
- Inhalation (aerosol liquid)

Common Uses
- Treatment of asthma and COPD

Quick Facts
- Prime inhaler prior to first use and when inhaler has not been used for more than 7 days by spraying into air 2 times. Shake inhaler well for 5 seconds before each use.
- Counsel patients to rinse mouth with water, without swallowing, after each use to prevent oral candidiasis.
- Side effects: headache, oral candidiasis, nasopharyngitis, upper or lower respiratory tract infection, allergic rhinitis, sinusitis

BUPRENORPHINE-NALOXONE

Brand Names
- Suboxone, Zubsolv, Bunavail

Pharmacologic Class
- Opioid agonist/antagonist

Mechanism of Action
- Buprenorphine is a partial agonist at the mu-opioid receptor and an antagonist at the kappa-opioid receptor. Naloxone is a mu-opioid receptor antagonist.

Dosage Forms
- Oral (sublingual tablet, sublingual film, buccal film)

Common Use
- Treatment of opioid dependence

Quick Facts
- DEA Schedule III
- Counsel patient not to chew, swallow, or move sublingual/buccal film after it is placed in mouth. Do not chew or swallow sublingual tablets.
- Use with caution in patients with decreased hepatic function. Use is not recommended in patients with severe hepatic impairment.
- Avoid abrupt discontinuation to prevent withdrawal symptoms.
- Side effects: headache, sweating, nausea, vomiting, constipation

BUPROPION

Brand Names
- Wellbutrin, Zyban

Pharmacologic Class
- Dopamine-norepinephrine reuptake inhibitor

Mechanism of Action
- Inhibits the neuronal uptake of dopamine and norepinephrine and blocks nicotinic acetylcholinergic receptors.

Dosage Form
- Oral (tablet)

Common Uses
- Treatment of depression and seasonal affective disorder; smoking cessation

Quick Facts
- Black Box Warning – Increased risk of suicidal thoughts and behavior, especially in children, adolescents, and young adults.
- Contraindicated in patients with a seizure disorder, current or prior diagnosis of bulimia or anorexia nervosa, during or within 14 days of MAOI administration.
- Do not exceed 450 mg/day due to seizure risk.
- If used for smoking cessation, start 1 week before target quit date.
- Side effects: dry mouth, insomnia, tremors, headache

BUSPIRONE

Brand Name
- Buspar

Pharmacologic Class
- Antianxiety agent

Mechanism of Action
- Majority of clinical effects believed to be due to its high affinity for serotonin 5-HT$_{1A}$ receptors.

Dosage Form
- Oral (tablet)

Common Use
- Treatment of anxiety

Quick Facts
- May take 2 to 4 weeks for optimal effect.
- Avoid alcohol, grapefruit, and grapefruit juice while taking medication.
- Avoid concomitant use with MAOIs.
- Use is not recommended in patients with severe hepatic or renal impairment.
- Can be taken with or without food but must be consistent.
- Side effects: nausea, dizziness, excitement, headache

CALCITRIOL (oral)

Brand Name
- Rocaltrol

Pharmacologic Class
- Vitamin D analog

Mechanism of Action
- Increases serum blood calcium levels by promoting absorption in the intestines, renal tubular reabsorption, and release from bone. It also suppresses the synthesis of parathyroid hormone.

Dosage Forms
- Oral (tablet, solution)

Common Uses
- Treatment of hypocalcemia in patients with hypoparathyroidism and pseudohypoparathyroidism, hypocalcemia in patients on chronic renal dialysis, and secondary hyperparathyroidism in patients with chronic kidney disease

Quick Facts
- Patients should be counseled to report signs or symptoms of hypercalcemia, which include dry mouth, weakness, headache, constipation, nausea, vomiting, and arthralgia
- Drink plenty of fluids when using oral form.
- Counsel patients to maintain adequate intake of calcium and to avoid additional vitamin D supplements.
- Side effects with high doses include hypercalcemia, nausea, constipation, loss of appetite

CARBAMAZEPINE

Brand Names
- Tegretol, Carbatrol, Epitol, Equetro

Pharmacologic Class
- Anticonvulsant

Mechanism of Action
- Mechanism of action remains unknown. In animals, it appears to prevent seizures by reducing polysynaptic responses and blocking the post-tetanic potentiation.

Dosage Forms
- Oral (tablet, chewable tablet, capsule, suspension)

Common Uses
- Treatment of epilepsy (partial, generalized, and mixed types), bipolar disorder, and trigeminal neuralgia

Quick Facts
- Black Box Warnings – Serious and sometimes fatal dermatologic reactions including toxic epidermal necrolysis and Stevens-Johnson syndrome can occur, especially in patients with the HLA-B*1502 gene who are almost exclusively of Asian ancestry. Aplastic anemia and agranulocytosis have also been reported.
- Potent CYP450 inducer and autoinducer.
- Side effects: dizziness, drowsiness, ataxia, nausea, vomiting

CARBIDOPA-LEVODOPA

Brand Names
- Sinemet, Duopa, Rytary

Pharmacologic Class
- Antiparkinson agent

Mechanism of Action
- Levodopa crosses the blood-brain barrier and is converted into dopamine. Carbidopa prevents the peripheral plasma breakdown of levodopa by inhibiting its decarboxylation.

Dosage Forms
- Oral (tablet, disintegrating tablet, suspension, capsule)

Common Uses
- Treatment of Parkinson's disease and parkinsonism

Quick Facts
- Avoid abrupt discontinuation due to potential for neuroleptic malignant syndrome-like symptoms.
- A wearing-off effect may occur at the end of a dosing interval.
- Counsel patients that medication may discolor urine, saliva, or sweat to a dark red, brown, or black color, which can stain clothing.
- Counsel patients that a change in diet to high-protein foods can decrease absorption. Iron can also decrease absorption.
- Side effects: nausea, dizziness, orthostasis, dyskinesias, confusion, hallucinations

CARISOPRODOL

Brand Name
- Soma

Pharmacologic Class
- Skeletal muscle relaxant

Mechanism of Action
- Mechanism of action is unknown. In animals, muscle relaxation is associated with blocking neuronal activity in the spinal cord and in the descending reticular formation of the brain.

Dosage Form
- Oral (tablet)

Common Use
- Treatment of discomfort associated with acute, painful musculoskeletal conditions

Quick Facts
- DEA Schedule IV
- Medication should be used for short periods (up to 2 or 3 weeks).
- Avoid concomitant use with alcohol and other CNS depressants.
- Counsel patients to report idiosyncratic symptoms, which include extreme weakness, vision loss, euphoria, and confusion.
- Use with caution in patients with hepatic or renal impairment.
- Side effects: drowsiness, headache, dizziness

CARVEDILOL

Brand Name
- Coreg

Pharmacologic Class
- $Beta_1$/$beta_2$-blocker and $alpha_1$-blocker

Mechanism of Action
- Blocks stimulation of $beta_1$ (myocardial) and $beta_2$ (pulmonary, vascular)-adrenergic receptors which reduces cardiac output, reduces exercise-induced tachycardia and/or isoproterenol-induced tachycardia, and reduces reflex orthostatic tachycardia. Blockade of $alpha_1$-adrenergic receptors causes vasodilation of blood vessels.

Dosage Form
- Oral (tablet)

Common Uses
- Treatment of hypertension, heart failure, and impaired left ventricular dysfunction following MI

Quick Facts
- Contraindications include bronchial asthma or related bronchial spastic condition, 2nd or 3rd degree AV block, decompensated heart failure requiring IV inotropic therapy, and severe bradycardia.
- Avoid abrupt discontinuation.
- Use with caution in patients with hepatic impairment.
- Take with food to decrease orthostatic hypotension.
- Side effects: hypotension, hyperglycemia, dizziness, fatigue

CEFDINIR

Brand Name
- Omnicef

Pharmacologic Class
- Cephalosporin antibiotic (3rd generation)

Mechanism of Action
- Inhibits bacterial cell wall synthesis by binding to one or more of the penicillin-binding proteins, which inhibits the final transpeptidation step of peptidoglycan synthesis in bacterial cell walls.

Dosage Forms
- Oral (tablet, powder for suspension)

Common Uses
- Treatment of acute otitis media, sinusitis, community-acquired pneumonia, skin and skin structure infections, acute exacerbation of chronic bronchitis, and pharyngitis/tonsillitis

Quick Facts
- Reduce dosage in renal impairment (CrCl < 30 mL/min).
- Do not take within 2 hours of aluminum or magnesium-containing antacids or iron supplements.
- Use with caution in patients with a history of penicillin allergy.
- Discard unused suspension 10 days after reconstitution.
- Side effects: diarrhea, abdominal pain, nausea, rash, hives

CEFUROXIME AXETIL

Brand Name
- Ceftin

Pharmacologic Class
- Cephalosporin antibiotic (2nd generation)

Mechanism of Action
- Inhibits bacterial cell wall synthesis by binding to one or more of the penicillin-binding proteins, which inhibits the final transpeptidation step of peptidoglycan synthesis in bacterial cell walls.

Dosage Forms
- Oral (tablet, powder for suspension)

Common Uses
- Treatment of acute otitis media, sinusitis, skin and skin structure infections, acute exacerbation of chronic bronchitis, pharyngitis/tonsillitis, impetigo, Lyme disease (early), and UTIs

Quick Facts
- Reduce dosage in renal impairment (CrCl < 30 mL/min).
- Use with caution in patients with a history of penicillin allergy.
- Administer suspension with food. Discard unused portion 10 days after reconstitution.
- Side effects: diarrhea, nausea, vomiting, rash, hives

CELECOXIB

Brand Name
- Celebrex

Pharmacologic Class
- COX-2 inhibitor

Mechanism of Action
- Prevents the synthesis of prostaglandins by inhibiting the cyclooxygenase-2 (COX-2) enzyme.

Dosage Form
- Oral (capsule)

Common Uses
- Treatment of osteoarthritis, rheumatoid arthritis, ankylosing spondylitis, and acute pain

Quick Facts
- Black Box Warning – Increased risk of cardiovascular thrombotic events and GI bleeding, ulceration, and perforation. Contraindicated in the setting of coronary artery bypass graft surgery.
- Contraindicated in patients with an allergy to sulfonamides.
- Pregnant patients should avoid use starting at 30 weeks gestation due to the risk of premature closure of the ductus arteriosus.
- Avoid in patients with severe renal or hepatic impairment.
- Side effects: dyspepsia, headache, abdominal pain, upper respiratory tract infection, diarrhea

CEPHALEXIN

Brand Name
- Keflex

Pharmacologic Class
- Cephalosporin antibiotic (1st generation)

Mechanism of Action
- Inhibits bacterial cell wall synthesis by binding to one or more of the penicillin-binding proteins which inhibits the final transpeptidation step of peptidoglycan synthesis in bacterial cell walls.

Dosage Forms
- Oral (tablet, capsule, powder for suspension)

Common Uses
- Treatment of otitis media, respiratory tract infections, UTIs, skin and skin structure infections, and bone infections

Quick Facts
- Reduce dosage in renal impairment (CrCl < 30 mL/min).
- Use with caution in patients with a history of penicillin allergy.
- Keep suspension refrigerated. Discard unused portion 14 days after reconstitution.
- Side effects: diarrhea, abdominal pain, rash, hives

CHLORHEXIDINE GLUCONATE (oral)

Brand Names
- Peridex, Paroex, Periogard

Pharmacologic Class
- Antibacterial

Mechanism of Action
- Disrupts the plasma membrane of the bacterial cell, causing leakage of the intracellular material and precipitation of cytoplasmic components.

Dosage Form
- Oral (solution)

Common Uses
- Treatment of gingivitis and periodontitis

Quick Facts
- Recommended use is to rinse twice daily for 30 seconds after brushing teeth, then expectorate.
- Do not rinse with water or other mouthwashes, brush teeth, or eat immediately after using.
- Side effects: staining of teeth, increase in calculus formation, altered taste perception

CHLORTHALIDONE

Brand Name
- Thalitone

Pharmacologic Class
- Thiazide diuretic

Mechanism of Action
- Inhibits sodium and chloride reabsorption in the renal distal convoluted tubule.

Dosage Form
- Oral (tablet)

Common Uses
- Treatment of hypertension and edema

Quick Facts
- Contraindicated in anuria.
- Should be taken in the morning with food.
- Patients should be monitored for hyponatremia, hypochloremic alkalosis, and hypokalemia.
- Patients should report symptoms of potassium loss, which include excess thirst, drowsiness, muscle pains or cramps, nausea, vomiting, increased heart rate or pulse.
- Side effects: orthostatic hypotension, dizziness, headache, hyperuricemia, pancreatitis

CHOLECALCIFEROL

Brand Name
- Delta D3

Pharmacologic Class
- Vitamin D analog

Mechanism of Action
- Cholecalciferol is converted to calcifediol in the liver, then to calcitriol in the kidney, which increases the absorption of calcium and phosphate in the intestines, the release of calcium from bone, and promotes the renal tubule reabsorption of calcium. Calcitriol also suppresses the synthesis of parathyroid hormone.

Dosage Forms
- Oral (tablet, capsule, solution, suspension)

Common Use
- Treatment of vitamin D deficiency

Quick Facts
- Patients should be counseled to report signs or symptoms of hypercalcemia, which include dry mouth, constipation, weakness, headache, arthralgia, nausea, and vomiting.
- Counsel patients to maintain adequate intake of calcium and to avoid additional vitamin D supplements.
- Side effects with high doses include hypercalcemia, nausea, constipation, loss of appetite

CIPROFLOXACIN (oral)

Brand Name
- Cipro

Pharmacologic Class
- Fluoroquinolone antibiotic

Mechanism of Action
- Prevents the synthesis of bacterial DNA by inhibiting DNA gyrase (topoisomerase II) and topoisomerase IV.

Dosage Forms
- Oral (tablet, powder for suspension), intravenous (solution)

Common Uses
- Treatment of lower respiratory tract infections, UTIs, sinusitis, skin and skin structure infections, bone and joint infections, gonorrhea, and infectious diarrhea

Quick Facts
- Black Box Warnings – Risk of tendinitis, tendon rupture, peripheral neuropathy, CNS effects, and exacerbation of myasthenia gravis.
- Take medication 2 hours before or 6 hours after aluminum or magnesium-containing antacids or products containing calcium, iron, or zinc.
- Potent CYP1A2 inhibitor.
- May cause QT prolongation.
- Drink plenty of fluids to prevent crystalluria.
- Side effects: nausea, rash, diarrhea, sun sensitivity

CIPROFLOXACIN-DEXAMETHASONE

Brand Name
- Ciprodex

Pharmacologic Class
- Combination fluoroquinolone antibiotic and cortico-steroid

Mechanism of Action
- Ciprofloxacin prevents the synthesis of bacterial DNA by inhibiting DNA gyrase (topoisomerase II) and topoisomerase IV. Dexamethasone suppresses inflammation by inhibiting inflammatory cells and the release of inflammatory mediators.

Dosage Form
- Otic (suspension)

Common Uses
- Treatment of acute otitis media and acute otitis externa

Quick Facts
- To instill drops, warm bottle in hands for 1 to 2 minutes, as cold suspension can cause dizziness. Shake bottle gently. Lie down or tilt head so that affected ear faces upward. Straighten the ear canal by pulling earlobe up and back for adults or down and back for children. Instill the prescribed number of drops into the ear canal. Keep the ear facing up for 60 seconds.
- Side effects: ear discomfort, ear pain, ear pruritis

CITALOPRAM

Brand Name
- Celexa

Pharmacologic Class
- SSRI

Mechanism of Action
- Inhibits the reuptake of serotonin in presynaptic neurons of the CNS.

Dosage Forms
- Oral (tablet, solution)

Common Use
- Treatment of depression

Quick Facts
- Black Box Warning – Increased risk of suicidal thoughts and behavior in children, adolescents, and young adults.
- Risk of dose-dependent QT interval prolongation. (Doses greater than 40 mg/day are not recommended.)
- May increase the risk of bleeding events. Concomitant use of aspirin, NSAIDs, warfarin and other anticoagulants can increase risk.
- Do not abruptly discontinue medication.
- Use is contraindicated during or within 14 days of MAOI administration.
- Patients should report symptoms of hyponatremia, which include headache, confusion, and weakness.
- Side effects: somnolence, insomnia, impotence, dry mouth, nausea

CLARITHROMYCIN

Brand Name
▪ Biaxin

Pharmacologic Class
▪ Macrolide antibiotic

Mechanism of Action
▪ Binds to the 50S subunit of the bacterial ribosome, which inhibits RNA-dependent protein synthesis.

Dosage Forms
▪ Oral (tablet, powder for suspension)

Common Uses
▪ Treatment of community-acquired pneumonia, acute otitis media, COPD exacerbations, skin and soft tissue infections, *H. pylori* infection, pharyngitis/tonsillitis, and mycobacterial infections

Quick Facts
▪ Reduce dosage by 50% in patients with CrCl < 30 mL/min.
▪ Take extended-release tablets with food.
▪ Can prolong the QT interval.
▪ Strong CYP3A4 inhibitor.
▪ Store suspension at room temperature and discard 14 days after reconstitution.
▪ Side effects: diarrhea, nausea, dysgeusia, abdominal pain, dyspepsia

CLINDAMYCIN (oral)

Brand Name
- Cleocin

Pharmacologic Class
- Lincosamide antibiotic

Mechanism of Action
- Binds to the 50S subunit of the bacterial ribosome, which inhibits protein synthesis.

Dosage Form
- Oral (capsule)

Common Uses
- Treatment of lower respiratory tract infections, skin and skin structure infections, intrabdominal infections, septicemia, and gynecological infections

Quick Facts
- Black Box Warning – Risk of *C. difficile*-associated diarrhea and severe colitis which may be fatal.
- Use with caution in the elderly, in patients with a history of gastrointestinal disease (particularly colitis), and in patients with severe hepatic disease.
- Take with a full glass of water to prevent esophageal irritation.
- Side effects: diarrhea, nausea, vomiting, rash

CLOBETASOL

Brand Names
- Clobex, Olux, Temovate

Pharmacologic Class
- Corticosteroid

Mechanism of Action
- Has anti-inflammatory, antipruritic, and vasoconstrictive properties. The anti-inflammatory effect is believed to be due to stimulation of phospholipase A_2 inhibitory proteins. These proteins subsequently block the release of arachidonic acid, which is a precursor to leukotrienes and prostaglandins.

Dosage Forms
- Topical (solution, cream, spray, shampoo, lotion, ointment, gel)

Common Uses
- Treatment of inflammatory and pruritic manifestations of corticosteroid-responsive dermatoses

Quick Facts
- Do not use for more than 2 consecutive weeks, as topical steroid overuse can cause thinning of the skin and striae.
- Do not use with bandages, wraps, or other occlusive dressings unless directed by prescriber.
- Apply sparingly and wash hands after application.
- Avoid contact with face, axillae, and groin.
- Side effects: pruritis, burning sensation, hypothalamic-pituitary-adrenal axis suppression

CLONAZEPAM

Brand Name
- Klonopin

Pharmacologic Class
- Benzodiazepine

Mechanism of Action
- Causes CNS depression by potentiating the effects of GABA (an inhibitory neurotransmitter).

Dosage Forms
- Oral (tablet, disintegrating tablet)

Common Uses
- Treatment of panic disorder and seizure disorders

Quick Facts
- DEA Schedule IV
- Black Box Warning – Concomitant use with opioids increases risk of sedation, respiratory depression, coma, or death.
- With long-term use, avoid abrupt discontinuation to prevent withdrawal symptoms.
- Contraindicated in patients with significant liver disease and acute narrow-angle glaucoma.
- Side effects: drowsiness, dizziness, ataxia

CLONIDINE

Brand Names
- Catapres, Kapvay

Pharmacologic Class
- Alpha$_2$-agonist

Mechanism of Action
- Stimulates alpha$_2$-adrenergic receptors in the brain, which reduces sympathetic outflow from the CNS to the heart, kidneys, and peripheral vasculature.

Dosage Forms
- Oral (tablet), transdermal (patch)

Common Uses
- Treatment of hypertension and ADHD (extended-release tablet)

Quick Facts
- Avoid abrupt discontinuation to prevent withdrawal symptoms, which include rebound hypertension, headache, tachycardia, nausea, and anxiety.
- Topical patches should be applied once weekly to a clean, hairless area of the upper outer arm or chest. If redness occurs a topical steroid may be applied to the area before application.
- Reduce dose in renal impairment.
- Side effects: dry mouth, drowsiness, headache, upper abdominal pain, impotence

CLOPIDOGREL

Brand Name
- Plavix

Pharmacologic Class
- $P2Y_{12}$ inhibitor

Mechanism of Action
- Inhibits the binding of ADP to its platelet $P2Y_{12}$ receptor which prevents activation of the GPIIb/IIIa complex and platelet aggregation.

Dosage Form
- Oral (tablet)

Common Uses
- Reduction of atherothrombotic events for patients with a history of recent MI, recent stroke, or established peripheral arterial disease; treatment of acute coronary syndrome

Quick Facts
- Black Box Warning – Effectiveness of medication will be diminished in patients that have reduced function of CYP2C19 (CYP2C19*2 and *3 alleles are nonfunctional).
- Rare cases of thrombotic thrombocytopenia purpura (TTP) have been reported. Symptoms include fever, fatigue, purplish bruises, and yellowing of the skin or eyes.
- Discontinue 5 days prior to elective surgery.
- Side effects: bleeding, bruising, rash, chest pain

CLOTRIMAZOLE-BETAMETHASONE

Brand Name
- Lotrisone

Pharmacologic Class
- Combination antifungal and corticosteroid

Mechanism of Action
- Clotrimazole decreases the synthesis of ergosterol, which is an essential component of fungal cell membranes. Betamethasone has anti-inflammatory, antipruritic, and vasoconstrictive properties. The anti-inflammatory effect is believed to be due to stimulation of phospholipase A_2 inhibitory proteins. These proteins subsequently block the release of arachidonic acid, which is a precursor to leukotrienes and prostaglandins.

Dosage Forms
- Topical (cream, lotion)

Common Use
- Treatment of fungal infections (tinea corporis, tinea cruris, tinea pedis)

Quick Facts
- Do not use with occlusive dressings.
- Do not apply to the face or axillae.
- Side effects: stinging, burning, peeling, irritation of the skin

COLCHICINE

Brand Names
- Colcrys, Mitigare, Gloperba

Pharmacologic Class
- Antigout agent

Mechanism of Action
- Blocks the inflammasome complex in neutrophils and monocytes that mediates activation of interleukin-1β, thus preventing the activation, degranulation, and migration of neutrophils.

Dosage Forms
- Oral (tablet, capsule, solution)

Common Uses
- Prophylaxis and treatment of gout; treatment of familial Mediterranean fever

Quick Facts
- The recommended dose for treatment of a gout flare is 1.2 mg at the first sign of the flare followed by 0.6 mg 1 hour later. Maximum recommended dose for treatment of gout flares is 1.8 mg over a 1 hour period.
- For gout flares, a treatment course should be repeated no more than once every 2 weeks.
- Bone marrow depression, agranulocytosis, aplastic anemia, and thrombocytopenia have been reported.
- Side effects: diarrhea, nausea, vomiting, abdominal pain

COLESEVELAM

Brand Name
- Welchol

Pharmacologic Class
- Bile acid sequestrant

Mechanism of Action
- Binds bile acids in the intestines to form a complex that is excreted in the feces, which causes increased oxidation of cholesterol to bile acid and lowers serum cholesterol.

Dosage Forms
- Oral (tablet, powder for suspension)

Common Uses
- Treatment of hyperlipidemia and adjunctive therapy for type 2 diabetes

Quick Facts
- Contraindicated in patients with serum triglyceride concentrations > 500 mg/dL, a history of hypertriglyceridemia-induced pancreatitis, or a history of bowel obstruction.
- May reduce the efficacy of oral contraceptives. Patients should take oral contraceptives at least 4 hours prior to taking colesevelam. Phenytoin, levothyroxine, glyburide, and vitamin supplements should also be taken 4 hours prior.
- Take tablets with food and a liquid.
- Side effects: constipation, indigestion, vomiting

CONJUGATED ESTROGENS

Brand Name
- Premarin

Pharmacologic Class
- Endocrine agent

Mechanism of Action
- Binds to nuclear receptors in estrogen-responsive tissues, and regulates gene transcription and formation of mRNA. Also reduces the levels of luteinizing hormone and follicle-stimulating hormone secreted by the pituitary gland through a negative feedback mechanism.

Dosage Forms
- Oral (tablet), vaginal (cream), intravenous (powder for solution)

Common Uses
- Treatment of vasomotor symptoms, vulvar and vaginal atrophy associated with menopause; prevention of postmenopausal osteoporosis; treatment of hypoestrogenism in females

Quick Facts
- Black Box Warnings – Estrogens increase the risk of endometrial cancer. Estrogens with or without progestins should not be used for the prevention of cardiovascular disease. Increased risks of MI, stroke, invasive breast cancer, pulmonary emboli, and DVT in postmenopausal women (50 to 79 years of age) using estrogens combined with progestins have been reported. An increased risk of developing probable dementia in postmenopausal women ≥ 65 years of age has been reported in women using estrogen alone or estrogen combined with progestins.
- Estrogens, with or without progestins, should be prescribed at the lowest effective doses and for the shortest duration possible.
- Side effects: cardiovascular or thromboembolic disorders, breast tenderness, headache, nausea

CONJUGATED ESTROGENS-MEDROXYPROGESTERONE

Brand Names
- Prempro, Premphase

Pharmacologic Class
- Estrogen and progestin combination

Mechanism of Action
- Estrogens modulate the pituitary secretion of the gonadotropins, luteinizing hormone, and follicle-stimulating hormone, through a negative feedback mechanism thereby reducing the elevated levels of these gonadotropins seen in postmenopausal women. Medroxyprogesterone converts a proliferative endometrium into a secretory one, reducing endometrial growth and the risk of endometrial carcinoma.

Dosage Form
- Oral (tablet)

Common Uses
- Treatment of vasomotor symptoms, vulvar and vaginal atrophy associated with menopause; prevention of postmenopausal osteoporosis

Quick Facts
- Black Box Warnings – Estrogens increase the risk of endometrial cancer. Estrogens with or without progestins should not be used for the prevention of cardiovascular disease. Increased risks of MI, stroke, invasive breast cancer, pulmonary emboli, and DVT in postmenopausal women (50 to 79 years of age) using estrogens combined with progestins have been reported. An increased risk of developing probable dementia in postmenopausal women ≥ 65 years of age has been reported in women using estrogen alone or estrogen combined with progestins.
- Estrogens, with or without progestins, should be prescribed at the lowest effective doses and for the shortest duration possible.
- Side effects: dysmenorrhea, depression, weight changes, breast tenderness, nausea

CYANOCOBALAMIN

Brand Names
- Vitamin B_{12}, Nasocobal

Pharmacologic Class
- Vitamin

Mechanism of Action
- An essential B-vitamin that is necessary for cell reproduction, growth, and synthesis of myelin and nucleoprotein. Also plays an important role in the metabolism of fats and carbohydrates.

Dosage Forms
- Oral (tablet, lozenge, disintegrating tablet, chewable tablet, solution), nasal (solution), injection solution (IM/IV)

Common Use
- Treatment of vitamin B_{12} deficiency

Quick Facts
- Vitamin B_{12}, hematocrit, reticulocyte count, folate and iron levels should be obtained before treatment.
- Extended-release tablets should be taken with food.
- Sublingual dosage forms should be left under tongue for 30 seconds before swallowing.
- Nasal spray should be administered at least 1 hour before or 1 hour after ingesting hot foods or liquids.
- Side effects: diarrhea, edema, itching, rash
- Side effects with intranasal use: headache, asthenia, paresthesia

CYCLOBENZAPRINE

Brand Names
- Flexeril, Amrix, Fexmid

Pharmacologic Class
- Skeletal muscle relaxant

Mechanism of Action
- Acts at the brain stem to reduce tonic somatic motor activity, influencing both gamma and alpha motor neurons leading to a reduction in muscle spasms.

Dosage Forms
- Oral (tablet, capsule)

Common Use
- Treatment of skeletal muscle spasm associated with acute, painful musculoskeletal conditions

Quick Facts
- Use is contraindicated during or within 14 days of MAOI administration.
- Use with caution in patients with narrow-angle glaucoma, increased intraocular pressure or urinary frequency/hesitancy due to anticholinergic effects.
- Reduce dosing in patients with hepatic impairment.
- May enhance the effects of alcohol, barbiturates, and other CNS depressants.
- Side effects: drowsiness, dry mouth, headache, abdominal pain, constipation, diarrhea

CYCLOSPORINE (ophthalmic)

Brand Names
- Restasis, Cequa

Pharmacologic Class
- Calcineurin inhibitor

Mechanism of Action
- Believed to act as a partial immune modulator in patients whose tear production is suppressed due to ocular inflammation associated with keratoconjunctivitis sicca (dry eye).

Dosage Forms
- Ophthalmic (emulsion, solution)

Common Use
- Treatment of dry eye that may be caused by inflammation

Quick Facts
- Patients should remove contact lenses prior to using. Lenses can be reinserted 15 minutes after administration. Allow at least 15 minutes between use of medication and artificial tears.
- Before using emulsion, invert unit dose vial a few times to obtain a uniform white opaque emulsion.
- Contents of single-use vial should be used immediately after opening, and remaining contents should be discarded after using.
- Side effects: ocular burning, blurred vision, eye pain, eye discharge

DABIGATRAN

Brand Name
- Pradaxa

Pharmacologic Class
- Direct thrombin inhibitor

Mechanism of Action
- Dabigatran and its active metabolites (acyl glucu-ronides) are competitive, direct thrombin inhibitors. They prevent thrombus development by inhibiting both free and clot-bound thrombin and thrombin-induced platelet aggregation.

Dosage Form
- Oral (capsule)

Common Uses
- Prevention of stroke and systemic embolism in patients with non-valvular atrial fibrillation; treatment and prevention of DVT and PE in patients who have been treated with a parenteral anticoagulant for 5 to 10 days; prevention of DVT and PE in patients who have undergone hip replacement surgery

Quick Facts
- Black Box Warning – Premature discontinuation increases the risk of thrombotic events. To reduce risk consider coverage with another anticoagulant if dabigatran is discontinued for a reason other than pathological bleeding or completion of therapy.
- Store medication in original container, and once opened use medication within 4 months.
- Side effects: gastritis, gastrointestinal hemorrhage, GERD

DESONIDE

Brand Names
- DesOwen, Desonate, Verdso

Pharmacologic Class
- Corticosteroid

Mechanism of Action
- Has anti-inflammatory, antipruritic, and vasoconstrictive properties. The anti-inflammatory effect is believed to be due to stimulation of phospholipase A_2 inhibitory proteins. These proteins subsequently block the release of arachidonic acid, which is a precursor to leukotrienes and prostaglandins.

Dosage Forms
- Topical (ointment, cream, gel, lotion, foam)

Common Uses
- Treatment of inflammatory and pruritic manifestations of corticosteroid-responsive dermatoses; treatment of atopic dermatitis

Quick Facts
- Do not use for more than 4 consecutive weeks.
- Do not use with bandages, wraps, or other occlusive dressings unless directed by prescriber.
- Apply sparingly and wash hands after application.
- Side effects: pruritis, burning sensation, hypothalamic-pituitary-adrenal axis suppression

DESVENLAFAXINE

Brand Name
- Pristiq

Pharmacologic Class
- SNRI

Mechanism of Action
- Increases the synaptic concentration of serotonin and norepinephrine in the CNS by inhibiting their reuptake at presynaptic nerve terminals.

Dosage Form
- Oral (tablet)

Common Use
- Treatment of depression

Quick Facts
- Black Box Warning – Increased risk of suicidal thoughts and behavior, especially in children, adolescents, and young adults.
- Do not abruptly discontinue medication.
- Symptomatic improvement may take several weeks.
- Use is contraindicated during or within 14 days of MAOI administration. Allow 7 days after stopping desvenlafaxine before starting an MAOI.
- Monitor blood pressure regularly.
- Side effects: nausea, dry mouth, constipation, hypertension, sweating, sexual dysfunction in men

DEXAMETHASONE (oral)

Brand Name
- Decadron

Pharmacologic Class
- Corticosteroid

Mechanism of Action
- Suppresses inflammation by inhibiting inflammatory cells and the release of inflammatory mediators.

Dosage Forms
- Oral (tablet, solution)

Common Uses
- Treatment of various allergic and inflammatory diseases, including endocrine disorders, respiratory diseases, and rheumatic disorders

Quick Facts
- Patients on long-term therapy should avoid live or live-attenuated vaccines due to drug-induced immunosuppression.
- Take with food to decrease GI upset.
- Contraindicated in patients with systemic fungal infections. (Infections may be exacerbated.)
- Has low sodium-retaining potential.
- Taper dose to prevent withdrawal symptoms if used longer than 2 weeks.
- Short-term side effects: insomnia, stomach upset, fluid retention, increased appetite
- Long-term side effects: Cushing's syndrome, osteoporosis, muscle wasting, growth suppression in children

DEXLANSOPRAZOLE

Brand Name
- Dexilant

Pharmacologic Class
- PPI

Mechanism of Action
- Suppresses gastric acid secretion by inhibiting the H^+/K^+-ATPase pump in parietal cells, blocking the final step of acid production.

Dosage Form
- Oral (capsule)

Common Uses
- Treatment of GERD and erosive esophagitis

Quick Facts
- Do not abruptly discontinue. Medication should be tapered to avoid acid rebound.
- Use with caution with other medications that require an acidic pH for absorption (itraconazole, ketoconazole, iron, etc.).
- Patients taking long-term should have adequate calcium and vitamin D intake. (Calcium citrate formulations will have improved absorption in basic pH.)
- Short-term side effects: headache, dizziness, diarrhea, constipation, upper respiratory tract infection
- Long-term side effects: increased risk of osteoporosis or fracture, vitamin B_{12} deficiency, hypomagnesemia

DEXMETHYLPHENIDATE

Brand Name
- Focalin

Pharmacologic Class
- CNS stimulant

Mechanism of Action
- Believed to block the reuptake of norepinephrine and dopamine in presynaptic nerve endings and increase their release into the extraneuronal space.

Dosage Forms
- Oral (tablet, capsule)

Common Use
- Treatment of ADHD

Quick Facts
- DEA Schedule II
- Black Box Warning – High potential for abuse, and administration for prolonged periods of time may lead to dependence. Misuse may cause sudden death and serious cardiovascular adverse reactions.
- Use is contraindicated during or within 14 days of MAOI administration.
- Gradually increase dosing and avoid abrupt discontinuation to prevent withdrawal symptoms.
- Can lower seizure threshold.
- Side effects: anorexia, weight loss, anxiety, nausea, dry mouth, headache

DIAZEPAM

Brand Names
- Valium, Diastat, Valtoco

Pharmacologic Class
- Benzodiazepine

Mechanism of Action
- Causes CNS depression by potentiating the effects of GABA (an inhibitory neurotransmitter).

Dosage Forms
- Oral (tablet, solution), nasal (spray), injection solution (IM/IV), rectal (gel)

Common Uses
- Treatment of anxiety disorders, alcohol withdrawal syndrome, muscle spasms, seizures, and status epilepticus

Quick Facts
- DEA Schedule IV
- Black Box Warning – Concomitant use with opioids increases risk of sedation, respiratory depression, coma, or death.
- Avoid abrupt discontinuation to prevent withdrawal symptoms.
- Avoid alcohol, grapefruit, and grapefruit juice while taking medication.
- Use with caution in patients with impaired renal or hepatic function.
- Side effects: drowsiness, dizziness, ataxia, headache

DICLOFENAC
(systemic and topical)

Brand Names
- Voltaren, Zorvolex

Pharmacologic Class
- NSAID

Mechanism of Action
- Prevents the synthesis of prostaglandins by inhibiting the cyclooxygenase-1 and cyclooxygenase-2 (COX-1 and 2) enzymes.

Dosage Forms
- Oral (tablet, capsule), topical (gel, patch, solution)

Common Uses
- Treatment of osteoarthritis pain, acute pain, and actinic keratosis

Quick Facts
- Black Box Warnings – Increased risk of cardiovascular thrombotic events and GI bleeding, ulceration, and perforation. Contraindicated in the setting of coronary artery bypass graft surgery.
- Contraindicated in patients with a history of asthma, urticaria, or other allergic-type reactions after taking aspirin or other NSAIDs.
- Pregnant patients should avoid use starting at 30 weeks gestation due to the risk of premature closure of the ductus arteriosus.
- Avoid in patients with severe renal or hepatic impairment.
- Side effects: dyspepsia, nausea, headache, edema, diarrhea, constipation

DICYCLOMINE

Brand Name
- Bentyl

Pharmacologic Class
- Anticholinergic

Mechanism of Action
- Blocks the action of acetylcholine at parasympathetic sites in smooth muscle, secretory gland tissue, and in the CNS.

Dosage Forms
- Oral (tablet, capsule, solution), intramuscular (solution)

Common Use
- Treatment of irritable bowel syndrome

Quick Facts
- Contraindications include GI or urinary tract obstruction, glaucoma, myasthenia gravis, reflux esophagitis, and use in infants < 6 months old.
- Use with caution in patients with renal impairment.
- Medication can cause anhidrosis – use caution during hot weather and with activities leading to an increase in core temperature or dehydration.
- Side effects: dry mouth, constipation, urinary retention, blurred vision

DIGOXIN

Brand Names
- Digitek, Digox, Lanoxin

Pharmacologic Class
- Antiarrhythmic agent

Mechanism of Action
- Inhibits the sodium-potassium ATPase pump in myocardial cells, which increases intracellular sodium and calcium concentrations, causing increased contractility of the heart. Digoxin also stimulates the parasympathetic nervous system via the vagus nerve, which decreases conduction velocity through the AV node, causing a slowing of the heart rate.

Dosage Forms
- Oral (tablet, solution), intravenous (solution)

Common Uses
- Treatment of heart failure and atrial fibrillation

Quick Facts
- Reduce dosage in renal impairment. (Dosage is based on CrCl and lean body weight.)
- Reduce dosage by 20 to 25% when changing from oral therapy to IV therapy.
- Risk of toxicity is increased in patients with hypokalemia, hypomagnesemia, or hypercalcemia.
- Patients should report symptoms of toxicity. First symptoms of toxicity include nausea, vomiting, and loss of appetite. Other symptoms of toxicity include arrhythmias, blurred or "yellow" vision, confusion, weakness, and abdominal pain.
- Side effects: diarrhea, nausea, vomiting, dizziness

DILTIAZEM

Brand Names
- Cardizem, Cartia XT, Dilacor XR, Tiazac

Pharmacologic Class
- Calcium channel blocker

Mechanism of Action
- Non-dihydropyridine CCB that blocks the transmembrane influx of calcium ions into vascular smooth muscle and cardiac muscle which results in increased peripheral arterial vasodilation and decreased peripheral vascular resistance. Also is a negative inotrope (decreased force) and negative chronotrope (decreased rate).

Dosage Forms
- Oral (tablet, capsule), intravenous (solution)

Common Uses
- Treatment of hypertension, atrial arrhythmia, paroxysmal supraventricular tachycardia, and chronic stable angina

Quick Facts
- Contraindications include hypotension (SBP < 90 mmHg), 2nd or 3rd degree AV block without a functioning pacemaker, and acute MI with pulmonary congestion on X-ray.
- Medication is both a substrate and inhibitor of CYP3A4.
- Do not abruptly discontinue medication.
- Side effects: peripheral edema, headache, dizziness, bradycardia

DIPHENOXYLATE-ATROPINE

Brand Name
- Lomotil

Pharmacologic Class
- Antidiarrheal

Mechanism of Action
- Diphenoxylate binds to intestinal opioid receptors in the enteric nervous system to block acetylcholine release and decrease peristalsis. Atropine has anticholinergic activity but is included in a subtherapeutic amount to discourage abuse.

Dosage Forms
- Oral (tablet, solution)

Common Use
- Treatment of diarrhea

Quick Facts
- DEA Schedule V
- Use is contraindicated in patients with diarrhea associated with enterotoxin-producing bacteria or pseudomembranous enterocolitis, and in patients with obstructive jaundice.
- Medication should be discontinued if clinical improvement of acute symptoms is not seen in 48 hours, and improvement of chronic symptoms is not seen within 10 days.
- Avoid use with alcohol and other CNS depressants.
- Side effects: drowsiness, abdominal pain, dizziness, euphoria

DIVALPROEX SODIUM

Brand Name
- Depakote

Pharmacologic Class
- Anticonvulsant

Mechanism of Action
- Divalproex dissociates to valproate in the GI tract. Its mechanism of action is unknown but is thought to be attributed to increased levels of GABA in the brain.

Dosage Forms
- Oral (tablet, capsule, solution), intravenous (solution)

Common Uses
- Treatment of simple, complex absence, and complex partial seizures, bipolar disorder; prevention of migraines

Quick Facts
- Black Box Warnings – Hepatic failure resulting in fatalities has occurred in patients, usually in the initial 6 months of therapy. Life-threatening pancreatitis has been reported. Valproate can cause major congenital malformations and neural tube defects, such as spina bifida.
- LFTs should be performed prior to therapy and at frequent intervals thereafter, especially during the first 6 months of treatment.
- Administer oral dosage forms with food to minimize GI upset.
- Side effects: alopecia, tremor, weight gain, nausea, thrombocytopenia

DONEPEZIL

Brand Name
- Aricept

Pharmacologic Class
- Cholinesterase inhibitor

Mechanism of Action
- Inhibits centrally-active acetylcholinesterase, which increases the amount of acetylcholine at cholinergic synapses.

Dosage Form
- Oral (tablet)

Common Use
- Treatment of Alzheimer's disease

Quick Facts
- Medication should be taken in the evening at bedtime.
- May be associated with QT prolongation. Also may have vagotonic effects on the heart which may manifest as bradycardia or heart block.
- Medication may increase gastric acid secretion. Use with caution in patients at risk of ulcer disease or with concomitant NSAID use.
- Likely to exaggerate succinylcholine-type muscle relaxation during anesthesia.
- Use with caution in patients with asthma or obstructive pulmonary disease.
- Side effects: diarrhea, nausea, vomiting, loss of appetite

DORZOLAMIDE-TIMOLOL

Brand Name
▪ Cosopt

Pharmacologic Class
▪ Combination carbonic anhydrase inhibitor and beta-blocker

Mechanism of Action
▪ Dorzolamide and timolol decrease intraocular pressure by reducing aqueous humor production.

Dosage Form
▪ Ophthalmic (solution)

Common Uses
▪ Treatment of open-angle glaucoma and ocular hypertension

Quick Facts
▪ Contraindications include active or history of bronchial asthma, 2nd or 3rd degree AV block, severe COPD, and sinus bradycardia.
▪ Systemic absorption is reduced when using nasolacrimal occlusion or closing the eyelids for 2 minutes after administration.
▪ Remove contact lenses before instilling medication and allow at least 15 minutes before reinserting.
▪ Wait at least 10 minutes after administration before using other ophthalmic medications.
▪ Side effects: burning, stinging, or itching of eyes, blurred vision, dysgeusia

DOXAZOSIN

Brand Name
- Cardura

Pharmacologic Class
- Alpha$_1$-blocker

Mechanism of Action
- Antagonist of alpha$_1$-adrenergic receptors, which decreases systemic vascular resistance and relaxes the smooth muscle of the prostate and bladder neck.

Dosage Form
- Oral (tablet)

Common Uses
- Treatment of hypertension and BPH

Quick Facts
- To avoid first-dose syncope, administer first dose of immediate-release tablets at bedtime and do not exceed 1 mg.
- If medication is discontinued for several days or a patient misses several doses, therapy should be re-started using the initial dosing regimen.
- Extended-release tablets should be taken with breakfast.
- Use is not recommended in patients with severe hepatic impairment.
- Side effects: orthostatic hypotension, dizziness, fatigue, headache

DOXEPIN (systemic)

Brand Name
- Silenor

Pharmacologic Class
- Tricyclic antidepressant

Mechanism of Action
- Increases the synaptic concentration of serotonin and norepinephrine in the CNS by inhibiting their reuptake at presynaptic nerve terminals. Also has histamine H_1 and H_2 receptor antagonist activity.

Dosage Forms
- Oral (tablet, capsule, solution)

Common Uses
- Treatment of depression, anxiety, and insomnia

Quick Facts
- Black Box Warning – Increased risk of suicidal thoughts and behavior in children, adolescents, and young adults.
- Can prolong the QT interval.
- Use is contraindicated during or within 14 days of MAOI administration.
- Do not abruptly discontinue medication.
- Avoid alcohol use.
- Side effects: dry mouth, nausea, constipation, dizziness, weight gain

DOXYCYCLINE

Brand Names
- Vibramycin, Monodox, Doryx, Oracea

Pharmacologic Class
- Tetracycline antibiotic

Mechanism of Action
- Inhibits bacterial protein synthesis by binding to the 30S ribosomal subunit.

Dosage Forms
- Oral (tablet, capsule, powder for suspension, syrup), intravenous (powder for solution)

Common Uses
- Treatment of respiratory tract infections, anthrax, gonorrhea, acne, rosacea, and malaria prophylaxis

Quick Facts
- Medication should be administered with at least 8 oz. of water to prevent esophageal irritation or ulceration and with food to prevent gastric irritation. (Oracea should be administered on an empty stomach 1 hour before or 2 hours after meals.)
- Medication can cause photosensitivity. Patients should use sunscreen and avoid prolonged exposure to sunlight and tanning beds.
- Can cause permanent discoloration of teeth and should not be used during tooth development (last half of pregnancy, infancy, and children ≤ 8 years old).
- Avoid concomitant oral use with iron, bismuth subsalicylate, or antacids containing aluminum, calcium, or magnesium.
- Side effects: diarrhea, nausea, rash

DULOXETINE

Brand Name
- Cymbalta

Pharmacologic Class
- SNRI

Mechanism of Action
- Increases the synaptic concentration of serotonin and norepinephrine in the CNS by inhibiting their reuptake at presynaptic nerve terminals. Also weakly inhibits the reuptake of dopamine.

Dosage Form
- Oral (capsule)

Common Uses
- Treatment of depression, generalized anxiety disorder, fibromyalgia, chronic musculoskeletal pain, and diabetic peripheral neuropathy

Quick Facts
- Black Box Warning – Increased risk of suicidal thoughts and behavior, especially in children, adolescents, and young adults.
- Do not abruptly discontinue medication.
- Symptomatic improvement may take several weeks.
- Use is contraindicated during or within 14 days of MAOI administration, and allow 5 days after stopping duloxetine before starting an MAOI.
- Monitor blood pressure regularly.
- Side effects: nausea, dry mouth, constipation, hypertension, sweating, sexual dysfunction in men

DUTASTERIDE

Brand Name
- Avodart

Pharmacologic Class
- 5-alpha reductase inhibitor

Mechanism of Action
- Inhibits both type I and type II isoforms of the 5-alpha reductase enzyme, which blocks the conversion of testosterone to dihydrotestosterone.

Dosage Form
- Oral (capsule)

Common Use
- Treatment of BPH

Quick Facts
- Medication should not be handled by women who are or may be pregnant because absorption through the skin may harm a male fetus.
- Patients should not donate blood for at least 6 months after last dose to prevent exposure to a pregnant transfusion recipient.
- Use with caution with concomitant use of potent, chronic CYP3A4 inhibitors.
- New baseline PSA level should be established after 3 to 6 months of treatment and the value doubled to compare with normal values in untreated men.
- Side effects: decreased libido, impotence, gynecomastia

ENALAPRIL

Brand Names
- Vasotec, Epaned

Pharmacologic Class
- ACE inhibitor

Mechanism of Action
- Inhibits the angiotensin converting enzyme (ACE), which prevents the conversion of angiotensin I to angiotensin II, a potent vasoconstrictor.

Dosage Forms
- Oral (tablet, solution)

Common Uses
- Treatment of hypertension and heart failure

Quick Facts
- Black Box Warning – Discontinue use as soon as possible if pregnancy is detected.
- Use caution in patients with impaired renal function.
- Patients should avoid potassium supplements or salt substitutes containing potassium without first consulting healthcare provider.
- Contraindicated in patients with a history of angioedema, concomitant use with aliskiren in diabetic patients, concomitant use with neprilysin inhibitor, or within 36 hours of switching to or from a neprilysin inhibitor
- Side effects: cough, headache, dizziness, hyperkalemia, angioedema

ENOXAPARIN

Brand Name
- Lovenox

Pharmacologic Class
- Anticoagulant

Mechanism of Action
- Low molecular weight heparin, which binds to and accelerates the activity of antithrombin III, which inhibits coagulation factor Xa and, to a lesser extent, factor IIa.

Dosage Form
- Injection solution (SubQ/IV)

Common Uses
- Prophylaxis of DVT in abdominal surgery, hip replacement surgery, knee replacement surgery, or medical patients with severely restricted mobility during acute illness; inpatient treatment of acute DVT with or without PE; outpatient treatment of acute DVT without PE; prophylaxis of ischemic complications of unstable angina and non-Q-wave MI; treatment of acute ST-segment elevation MI (STEMI)

Quick Facts
- Black Box Warning – Patients undergoing neuroaxial anesthesia or spinal puncture have an increased risk of epidural or spinal hematomas which could result in permanent paralysis.
- When administering enoxaparin, patients should be counseled to not expel the air bubble in the syringe prior to injection and to insert the needle at a 90-degree angle. They should rotate injection sites and avoid rubbing the site of injection as this will worsen bruising.
- Side effects: bleeding, anemia, thrombocytopenia, increased LFTs, nausea, diarrhea

EPINEPHRINE (IM/SubQ)

Brand Names
- EpiPen, Auvi-Q

Pharmacologic Class
- Sympathomimetic agent

Mechanism of Action
- Nonselective alpha- and beta-adrenergic receptor agonist. Through its action on alpha-adrenergic receptors, it reduces vasodilation and increases vascular permeability that occurs during anaphylaxis. Its action on beta-adrenergic receptors results in bronchial smooth muscle relaxation, which helps alleviate bronchospasm, wheezing, and dyspnea that may occur during anaphylaxis. Epinephrine also has relaxer effects on the smooth muscle of the stomach, intestine, uterus, and urinary bladder.

Dosage Form
- Injection solution (IM/SubQ)

Common Uses
- Treatment of type I allergic reactions, idiopathic anaphylaxis, and exercise-induced anaphylaxis

Quick Facts
- Inject intramuscularly or subcutaneously into anterolateral aspect of the thigh, through clothing if necessary.
- Do not inject into buttock. Injection into the buttock may not provide effective treatment of anaphylaxis and has been associated with Clostridial infections (gas gangrene).
- Injection solution should be clear, colorless, and free of particulate matter.
- Side effects: sweating, palpitations, headache, tremor, anxiety

EPOETIN ALFA

Brand Names
- Epogen, Procrit

Pharmacologic Class
- Hematopoietic agent

Mechanism of Action
- Stimulates the production of red blood cells by promoting the division and differentiation of committed erythroid progenitors in the bone marrow.

Dosage Form
- Injection solution (SubQ/IV)

Common Uses
- Treatment of anemia due to chronic kidney disease, chemotherapy, or zidovudine in patients with HIV-infection, and reduction of allogeneic RBC transfusions in patients undergoing elective noncardiac nonvascular surgery

Quick Facts
- Black Box Warnings – In chronic kidney disease, patients are at a greater risk for death and serious cardiovascular events and stroke when administered erythropoiesis-stimulating agents (ESAs) to target hemoglobin levels ≥ 11 g/dL. In cancer patients with certain tumor types (breast, non-small cell lung, head and neck, lymphoid, cervical), ESAs shorted overall survival and/or increased the risk of tumor progression or recurrence. When epoetin alfa is used preoperatively, DVT prophylaxis should be considered.
- Contraindicated in patients with uncontrolled hypertension.
- Do not shake medication vial because it may denature the glycoprotein and make it biologically inactive.
- Store medication in refrigerator.
- IV route is recommended for patients on hemodialysis.
- Side effects: hypertension, arthralgia, muscle spasm, headache, nausea

ERGOCALCIFEROL

Brand Names
- Drisdol, Calciferol

Pharmacologic Class
- Vitamin D analog

Mechanism of Action
- Promotes calcium and phosphate absorption in the small intestine, the release of calcium and phosphate from bone, and renal tubule reabsorption of calcium and phosphate.

Dosage Forms
- Oral (tablet, capsule, solution)

Common Uses
- Treatment of vitamin D deficiency, rickets, hypoparathyroidism, and hypophosphatemia

Quick Facts
- Patients should be counseled to report signs or symptoms of hypercalcemia, which include dry mouth, constipation, weakness, headache, arthralgia, nausea, and vomiting.
- May be taken without regard to food, but it is better absorbed when taken with foods containing fat.
- Counsel patients to maintain adequate intake of calcium and to avoid additional vitamin D supplements.
- Side effects with high doses include hypercalcemia, nausea, constipation, loss of appetite

ERYTHROMYCIN
(systemic and ophthalmic)

Brand Names
- Erythrocin, Ery-Tab

Pharmacologic Class
- Macrolide antibiotic

Mechanism of Action
- Binds to the 50S subunit of the bacterial ribosome, which inhibits RNA-dependent protein synthesis.

Dosage Forms
- Oral (tablet, capsule, powder for suspension), intravenous (powder for solution), ophthalmic (ointment)

Common Uses
- Treatment of respiratory tract infections, skin and soft tissue infections, pertussis, and ocular infections involving the conjunctiva or cornea

Quick Facts
- Administer base, PCE, or stearate dosage forms on an empty stomach (2 hours before or after a meal). Administer ethylsuccinate or delayed-release dosage forms without regard to meals.
- Oral forms can prolong the QT interval and are strong CYP3A4 inhibitors.
- For ophthalmic ointment, apply approximately a 1 cm ribbon to affected eye(s) up to 6 times daily.
- Side effects of oral forms: diarrhea, nausea, vomiting, abdominal pain, anorexia
- Side effects of ophthalmic ointment: eye irritation, redness

ESCITALOPRAM

Brand Name
- Lexapro

Pharmacologic Class
- SSRI

Mechanism of Action
- Inhibits the reuptake of serotonin in presynaptic neurons of the CNS.

Dosage Forms
- Oral (tablet, solution)

Common Uses
- Treatment of depression and generalized anxiety disorder

Quick Facts
- Black Box Warning – Increased risk of suicidal thoughts and behavior in children, adolescents, and young adults.
- Risk of dose-dependent QT interval prolongation.
- May increase the risk of bleeding events. Concomitant use of aspirin, NSAIDs, warfarin and other anticoagulants can increase risk.
- Do not abruptly discontinue medication.
- Use is contraindicated during or within 14 days of MAOI administration.
- Patients should report symptoms of hyponatremia, which include headache, confusion, and weakness.
- Side effects: somnolence, insomnia, impotence, dry mouth, nausea

ESOMEPRAZOLE

Brand Name
- Nexium

Pharmacologic Class
- PPI

Mechanism of Action
- Suppresses gastric acid secretion by inhibiting the H^+/K^+-ATPase pump in parietal cells, blocking the final step of acid production.

Dosage Forms
- Oral (capsule, tablet, powder for suspension), intravenous (powder for solution)

Common Uses
- Treatment of GERD, erosive esophagitis, Zollinger-Ellison syndrome, and *H. pylori* eradication; prevention of NSAID-associated gastric ulcers

Quick Facts
- Take at least 60 minutes before eating.
- Do not abruptly discontinue. Medication should be tapered to avoid acid rebound.
- Strong CYP2C19 inhibitor.
- Use with caution with other medications that require an acidic pH for absorption (itraconazole, ketoconazole, iron, etc.).
- Patients taking long-term should have adequate calcium and vitamin D intake. (Calcium citrate formulations are preferred.)
- Short-term side effects: headache, dry mouth, diarrhea, constipation, abdominal pain
- Long-term side effects: increased risk of osteoporosis or fracture, vitamin B_{12} deficiency, hypomagnesemia

ESTRADIOL

Brand Names
- Estrace, Climara, EstroGel

Pharmacologic Class
- Endocrine agent

Mechanism of Action
- Binds to nuclear receptors in estrogen-responsive tissues and regulates gene transcription and formation of mRNA. Also reduces the levels of luteinizing hormone and follicle-stimulating hormone secreted by the pituitary gland through a negative feedback mechanism.

Dosage Forms
- Oral (tablet), transdermal (gel, patch, solution), vaginal (ring, cream, tablet, capsule), intramuscular (oil)

Common Uses
- Treatment of vasomotor symptoms, vulvar and vaginal atrophy associated with menopause; prevention of postmenopausal osteoporosis; treatment of hypoestrogenism in females

Quick Facts
- Black Box Warnings – Estrogens increase the risk of endometrial cancer. Estrogens with or without progestins should not be used for the prevention of cardiovascular disease. Increased risks of MI, stroke, invasive breast cancer, pulmonary emboli, and DVT in postmenopausal women (50 to 79 years of age) using estrogens combined with progestins have been reported. An increased risk of developing probable dementia in postmenopausal women ≥ 65 years of age has been reported in women using estrogen alone or estrogen combined with progestins.
- Estrogens, with or without progestins, should be prescribed at the lowest effective doses and for the shortest duration possible.
- Side effects: cardiovascular or thromboembolic disorders, breast tenderness, headache, nausea

ESZOPICLONE

Brand Name
- Lunesta

Pharmacologic Class
- Hypnotic

Mechanism of Action
- Increases the activity of GABA by selective agonism at the benzodiazepine-1 receptor.

Dosage Form
- Oral (tablet)

Common Use
- Treatment of insomnia

Quick Facts
- DEA Schedule IV
- Black Box Warning – Complex sleep behaviors including sleep-walking, sleep-driving, and engaging in other activities while not fully awake may occur. Discontinue medication immediately if a patient experiences a complex sleep behavior. Use is contraindicated in patients who have experienced these events.
- Administer medication immediately before bedtime. Do not take with or immediately following a meal, as it may delay onset.
- Avoid alcohol and other CNS depressants.
- Side effects: headache, dysgeusia, dizziness, respiratory tract infection

ETANERCEPT

Brand Name
- Enbrel

Pharmacologic Class
- TNFα inhibitor

Mechanism of Action
- Binds to TNFα and prevents its interaction with cell surface TNF receptors, thereby inhibiting cytokine-driven inflammatory processes.

Dosage Forms
- Subcutaneous (solution, powder for solution)

Common Uses
- Treatment of rheumatoid arthritis, psoriatic arthritis, and plaque psoriasis

Quick Facts
- Black Box Warning – Patients are at an increased risk of serious infections leading to hospitalization or death, including tuberculosis (TB), bacterial sepsis, invasive fungal infections, and infections due to other opportunistic pathogens. Lymphoma and other malignancies have been reported.
- Avoid live vaccines during therapy.
- All patients should be screened for TB before and during therapy.
- Side effects: injection site pain or reaction, rash, upper respiratory tract infection, diarrhea

ETHINYL ESTRADIOL-DESOGESTREL

Brand Names
- Apri, Kariva, Mircette

Pharmacologic Class
- Oral contraceptive

Mechanism of Action
- Suppresses the production of luteinizing hormone and follicle-stimulating hormone, which prevents ovulation, and alters cervical mucus and the endometrial lining.

Dosage Form
- Oral (tablet)

Common Use
- Prevention of pregnancy

Quick Facts
- Black Box Warning – Cigarette smoking increases the risk of serious cardiovascular side effects from oral contraceptive use. Risk increases with age (> 35 years old) and heavy smoking (15 or more cigarettes per day).
- Contraindications include thromboembolic disorders, breast cancer, endometrial cancer, and severe hypertension.
- Medications that decrease the effectiveness of ethinyl estradiol-desogestrel include rifampin and St. John's wort.
- Take medication at the same time every day with no more than 24 hours between doses.
- Side effects: headache, nausea, breast tenderness, fatigue

ETHINYL ESTRADIOL-DROSPIRENONE

Brand Names
- Yaz, Yasmin, Ocella

Pharmacologic Class
- Oral contraceptive

Mechanism of Action
- Suppresses the production of luteinizing hormone and follicle-stimulating hormone, which prevents ovulation, and alters cervical mucus and the endometrial lining.

Dosage Form
- Oral (tablet)

Common Use
- Prevention of pregnancy

Quick Facts
- Black Box Warning – Cigarette smoking increases the risk of serious cardiovascular side effects from oral contraceptive use. Risk increases with age (> 35 years old) and heavy smoking (15 or more cigarettes per day).
- Contraindications include thromboembolic disorders, breast cancer, hepatic or renal dysfunction, and adrenal insufficiency.
- Drospirenone has antimineralocorticoid activity and can increase the risk of hyperkalemia.
- Medications that decrease the effectiveness of ethinyl estradiol-drospirenone include rifampin and St. John's wort.
- Take medication at the same time every day.
- Side effects: headache, nausea, breast tenderness, edema

ETHINYL ESTRADIOL-ETONOGESTREL

Brand Names
- NuvaRing, EluRyng

Pharmacologic Class
- Oral contraceptive

Mechanism of Action
- Suppresses the production of luteinizing hormone and follicle-stimulating hormone, which prevents ovulation, and alters cervical mucus and the endometrial lining.

Dosage Form
- Vaginal insert

Common Use
- Prevention of pregnancy

Quick Facts
- Black Box Warning – Cigarette smoking increases the risk of serious cardiovascular side effects from oral contraceptive use. Risk increases with age (> 35 years old) and heavy smoking (15 or more cigarettes per day).
- Contraindications include thromboembolic disorders, breast cancer, and severe hypertension.
- Medications that decrease the effectiveness of ethinyl estradiol-etonogestrel include rifampin and St. John's wort.
- Ring must remain in place for 3 consecutive weeks, then removed for 1 week.
- Medication should be refrigerated prior to dispensing. After dispensing, medication can be stored at room temperature for up to 4 months.
- Side effects: headache, nausea, breast tenderness

ETHINYL ESTRADIOL-LEVONORGESTREL

Brand Names
- Aviane, Alesse

Pharmacologic Class
- Oral contraceptive

Mechanism of Action
- Suppresses the production of luteinizing hormone and follicle-stimulating hormone, which prevents ovulation, and alters cervical mucus and the endometrial lining.

Dosage Form
- Oral (tablet)

Common Use
- Prevention of pregnancy

Quick Facts
- Black Box Warning – Cigarette smoking increases the risk of serious cardiovascular side effects from oral contraceptive use. Risk increases with age (> 35 years old) and heavy smoking (15 or more cigarettes per day).
- Contraindications include thromboembolic disorders, breast cancer, endometrial cancer, and severe hypertension.
- Medications that decrease the effectiveness of ethinyl estradiol-levonorgestrel include rifampin and St. John's wort.
- Take medication at the same time every day with no more than 24 hours between doses.
- Side effects: headache, nausea, breast tenderness, edema

ETHINYL ESTRADIOL-NORETHINDRONE

Brand Names
- Loestrin, Nortrel, Ortho-Novum

Pharmacologic Class
- Oral contraceptive

Mechanism of Action
- Suppresses the production of luteinizing hormone and follicle-stimulating hormone, which prevents ovulation, and alters cervical mucus and the endometrial lining.

Dosage Form
- Oral (tablet)

Common Use
- Prevention of pregnancy

Quick Facts
- Black Box Warning – Cigarette smoking increases the risk of serious cardiovascular side effects from oral contraceptive use. Risk increases with age (> 35 years old) and heavy smoking (15 or more cigarettes per day).
- Contraindications include thromboembolic disorders, breast cancer, endometrial cancer, and severe hypertension.
- Medications that decrease the effectiveness of ethinyl estradiol-norethindrone include rifampin and St. John's wort.
- Take medication at the same time every day with no more than 24 hours between doses.
- Side effects: headache, nausea, breast tenderness, edema

ETHINYL ESTRADIOL-NORGESTIMATE

Brand Names
- Ortho Tri-Cyclen, Previfem

Pharmacologic Class
- Oral contraceptive

Mechanism of Action
- Suppresses the production of luteinizing hormone and follicle-stimulating hormone, which prevents ovulation, and alters cervical mucus and the endometrial lining.

Dosage Form
- Oral (tablet)

Common Use
- Prevention of pregnancy

Quick Facts
- Black Box Warning – Cigarette smoking increases the risk of serious cardiovascular side effects from oral contraceptive use. Risk increases with age (> 35 years old) and heavy smoking (15 or more cigarettes per day).
- Contraindications include thromboembolic disorders, breast cancer, and severe hypertension.
- Medications that decrease the effectiveness of ethinyl estradiol-norgestimate include rifampin and St. John's wort.
- Take medication at the same time every day.
- Side effects: headache, nausea, breast tenderness, edema

ETODOLAC

Brand Name
- Lodine

Pharmacologic Class
- NSAID

Mechanism of Action
- Prevents the synthesis of prostaglandins by inhibiting the cyclooxygenase-1 and cyclooxygenase-2 (COX-1 and 2) enzymes.

Dosage Forms
- Oral (tablet, capsule)

Common Uses
- Treatment of acute pain (immediate release only), osteoarthritis, rheumatoid arthritis, and juvenile arthritis (extended release only)

Quick Facts
- Black Box Warnings – Increased risk of cardiovascular thrombotic events and GI bleeding, ulceration, and perforation. Contraindicated in the setting of coronary artery bypass graft surgery.
- Contraindicated in patients with a history of asthma, urticaria, or other allergic-type reactions after taking aspirin or other NSAIDs.
- Pregnant patients should avoid use starting in the third trimester due to the risk of premature closure of the ductus arteriosus.
- Avoid in patients with severe renal or hepatic impairment.
- Side effects: dyspepsia, nausea, edema, diarrhea, abdominal pain

EXENATIDE

Brand Names
- Bydureon, Byetta

Pharmacologic Class
- GLP-1 receptor agonist

Mechanism of Action
- Analog of incretin (glucagon-like peptide 1), which increases insulin secretion, decreases glucagon secretion, slows gastric emptying, and decreases food intake.

Dosage Forms
- Subcutaneous (solution, suspension)

Common Use
- Treatment of type 2 diabetes

Quick Facts
- Black Box Warning – Exenatide extended-release (Bydureon) causes an increased incidence of thyroid C-cell tumors in rats. The human relevance has not been determined. Exenatide extended-release is contraindicated in patients with a personal or family history of medullary thyroid carcinoma or in patients with Multiple Endocrine Neoplasia syndrome type 2 (MEN 2).
- Refrigerate unused syringes/vials. Used syringes/vials can be stored at room temperature for up to 30 days.
- Administer twice-daily formulation within 60 minutes before morning and evening meals.
- Use is not recommended in patients with severe renal impairment (CrCl < 30 mL/min).
- May cause acute pancreatitis.
- Side effects: nausea, headache, vomiting, diarrhea, and injection site pruritis and/or reaction

EZETIMIBE

Brand Name
- Zetia

Pharmacologic Class
- Antihyperlipidemic

Mechanism of Action
- Inhibits the absorption of cholesterol at the brush border of the small intestine, which decreases the delivery of cholesterol to the liver, reduces hepatic cholesterol stores, and increases the clearance of cholesterol from the blood.

Dosage Form
- Oral (tablet)

Common Use
- Treatment of hyperlipidemia

Quick Facts
- Patients also taking a bile acid sequestrant should take ezetimibe at least 2 hours before or 4 hours after the bile acid sequestrant.
- Patients should report symptoms of myopathy and rhabdomyolysis, which include muscle pain, tenderness, or weakness.
- Avoid use in moderate or severe hepatic impairment.
- Side effects: diarrhea, arthralgia, sinusitis, upper respiratory tract infection, pain in extremities

FAMOTIDINE

Brand Name
- Pepcid

Pharmacologic Class
- H_2 receptor antagonist

Mechanism of Action
- Inhibits histamine at H_2 receptors on gastric parietal cells, suppressing the concentration and volume of gastric acid secretion.

Dosage Forms
- Oral (tablet, powder for suspension), intravenous (solution)

Common Uses
- Treatment of GERD, erosive esophagitis, and peptic ulcer disease

Quick Facts
- Reduce dosage in renal impairment.
- Onset of action occurs within 1 hour and lasts approximately 10 to 12 hours.
- Discard unused suspension 30 days after reconstitution.
- Administer once daily (before bedtime) or twice daily (in the morning and before bedtime) as directed.
- May be used concomitantly with antacids.
- Side effects: diarrhea, constipation, headache, dizziness

FEBUXOSTAT

Brand Name
- Uloric

Pharmacologic Class
- Xanthine oxidase inhibitor

Mechanism of Action
- Decreases the production of uric acid by inhibiting the action of xanthine oxidase.

Dosage Form
- Oral (tablet)

Common Use
- Treatment of hyperuricemia in patients with gout

Quick Facts
- Black Box Warning – Increased risk of cardiovascular death and all-cause mortality in patients treated with febuxostat compared to allopurinol. Febuxostat should only be used in patients who are not treated effectively or experience severe side effects with allopurinol.
- Monitor LFTs at baseline and periodically thereafter.
- Monitor serum uric acid levels 2 weeks after initiating therapy.
- Limit daily dose to 40 mg in patients with severe renal impairment (CrCl < 30 mL/min).
- Side effects: rash, arthralgia, diarrhea, nausea, precipitation of acute gout attacks

FELODIPINE

Brand Name
- Plendil

Pharmacologic Class
- Calcium channel blocker

Mechanism of Action
- Dihydropyridine CCB that blocks the transmembrane influx of calcium ions into vascular smooth muscle and cardiac muscle which results in increased peripheral arterial vasodilation and decreased peripheral vascular resistance.

Dosage Form
- Oral (tablet)

Common Use
- Treatment of hypertension

Quick Facts
- May worsen angina and increase the risk of MI after starting or increasing dose.
- Avoid grapefruit and grapefruit juice while taking medication.
- May cause gingival hyperplasia. Patients should practice good dental hygiene.
- Do not abruptly discontinue medication.
- Side effects: peripheral edema, flushing, headache, reflex tachycardia

FENOFIBRATE

Brand Names
- Tricor, Trilipix

Pharmacologic Class
- Fibric acid

Mechanism of Action
- Activates peroxisome proliferator activated receptor alpha (PPARα) which increases lipolysis, activates lipoprotein lipase, and reduces production of apoprotein C-III. This causes a lowering of VLDL and triglycerides and an increase in HDL.

Dosage Forms
- Oral (tablet, capsule)

Common Uses
- Treatment of hyperlipidemia and hypertriglyceridemia

Quick Facts
- Contraindicated in active liver disease, severe renal disease, gallbladder disease, and when breastfeeding.
- Avoid concomitant use with statins due to increased risk of myopathy and rhabdomyolysis.
- Patients should report symptoms of hepatitis, gallstones, pancreatitis, or a rash.
- Limit alcohol intake during therapy.
- Side effects: abdominal pain, dyspepsia, myopathy, rhinitis

FENTANYL

Brand Names
- Duragesic, Subsys, Ionsys

Pharmacologic Class
- Opioid analgesic

Mechanism of Action
- Binds to the mu opioid receptor, which reduces neuronal cell excitability and transmission of nociceptive impulses.

Dosage Forms
- Transdermal (patch), oral (tablet, lozenge, film, sublingual liquid), intranasal (solution), injection (solution)

Common Uses
- Treatment of acute and chronic pain (Indication varies by dosage form.)

Quick Facts
- DEA Schedule II
- Black Box Warnings – Serious, life-threatening, or fatal respiratory depression may occur. Concomitant use with benzodiazepines increases risk of sedation, respiratory depression, coma, or death. Concomitant use with CYP3A4 inhibitors, or discontinuation of CYP3A4 inducers, can result in a fatal overdose of fentanyl. Prolonged use of fentanyl during pregnancy can result in neonatal opioid withdrawal syndrome.
- Fentanyl patches are for use only in opioid-tolerant patients for the management of persistent, moderate to severe chronic pain that requires continuous, around-the-clock opioid administration for an extended period of time and cannot be managed by other means.
- Apply fentanyl transdermal patch to an intact area of skin. Hair should be clipped if necessary. Do not cover the patch with a bandage or heating pad. Patches should not be cut. Dispose of used patches by folding in half and flushing down the toilet.
- Side effects: hypoventilation, fatigue, nausea, vomiting, constipation

FIDAXOMICIN

Brand Name
- Dificid

Pharmacologic Class
- Macrolide antibiotic

Mechanism of Action
- Inhibits RNA synthesis by binding to RNA polymerases.

Dosage Form
- Oral (tablet)

Common Use
- Treatment of *C. difficile*-associated diarrhea (CDAD)

Quick Facts
- Fidaxomicin has minimal systemic absorption and is not effective for the treatment of other types of infections.
- Fidaxomicin is a treatment option for the initial episode of CDAD, first recurrence (if vancomycin was used for the initial episode), and for second or subsequent recurrences.
- Adult dosing is 200 mg twice daily with or without food for 10 days. Patients should be counseled to finish course of therapy.
- Side effects: nausea, vomiting, abdominal pain, GI hemorrhage, anemia, neutropenia

FINASTERIDE

Brand Names
- Propecia, Proscar

Pharmacologic Class
- 5-alpha reductase inhibitor

Mechanism of Action
- Inhibits the type II isoform of the 5-alpha reductase enzyme, which blocks the conversion of testosterone to dihydrotestosterone.

Dosage Form
- Oral (tablet)

Common Uses
- Treatment of BPH and male pattern hair loss

Quick Facts
- Medication should not be handled by women who are or may be pregnant because absorption through the skin may harm a male fetus.
- New baseline PSA level should be established after 6 months of treatment and any increase should be evaluated.
- For treatment of BPH, 6 months of therapy may be necessary for maximal efficacy. For treatment of male pattern hair loss, 3 months of therapy may be necessary for clinical improvement.
- Side effects: decreased libido, impotence, breast tenderness

FLUCONAZOLE

Brand Name
- Diflucan

Pharmacologic Class
- Antifungal

Mechanism of Action
- Decreases the synthesis of ergosterol, which is an essential component of fungal cell membranes.

Dosage Forms
- Oral (tablet, powder for suspension), intravenous (solution)

Common Uses
- Treatment of candidiasis (esophageal, oropharyngeal, peritoneal, urinary tract, vaginal) and systemic candidiasis

Quick Facts
- Medication should be used with caution in patients with liver dysfunction. Patients who develop abnormal LFTs during therapy should be monitored for the development of more severe hepatic injury.
- Strong inhibitor of CYP2C9 and 2C19, moderate inhibitor of CYP3A4.
- May prolong the QT interval.
- Side effects: headache, nausea, abdominal pain, dysgeusia

FLUOCINONIDE

Brand Names
- Lidex, Vanos

Pharmacologic Class
- Corticosteroid

Mechanism of Action
- Fluocinonide has anti-inflammatory, antipruritic, and vasoconstrictive properties. The anti-inflammatory effect is believed to be due to stimulation of phospholipase A_2 inhibitory proteins. These proteins subsequently block the release of arachidonic acid, which is a precursor to leukotrienes and prostaglandins.

Dosage Forms
- Topical (cream, gel, ointment, solution)

Common Uses
- Treatment of inflammatory and pruritic manifestations of corticosteroid-responsive dermatoses

Quick Facts
- Contact prescriber if no improvement is seen within 2 weeks.
- Topical steroid overuse can cause thinning of the skin and striae.
- Do not use with bandages, wraps, or other occlusive dressings unless directed by prescriber.
- Apply sparingly and wash hands after application.
- Higher strength fluocinonide (0.1%) should not be used on the face, groin, or axillae.
- Side effects: pruritis, burning sensation, hypothalamic-pituitary-adrenal axis suppression

FLUOXETINE

Brand Names
- Prozac, Sarafem

Pharmacologic Class
- SSRI

Mechanism of Action
- Inhibits the reuptake of serotonin in presynaptic neurons of the CNS.

Dosage Forms
- Oral (tablet, solution, syrup)

Common Uses
- Treatment of depression, obsessive-compulsive disorder, panic disorder, premenstrual dysphoric disorder, and bulimia nervosa

Quick Facts
- Black Box Warning – Increased risk of suicidal thoughts and behavior in children, adolescents, and young adults.
- Risk of QT interval prolongation.
- Potent CYP2D6 inhibitor.
- May increase the risk of bleeding events. Concomitant use of aspirin, NSAIDs, warfarin and other anticoagulants can increase risk.
- Do not abruptly discontinue medication.
- Use is contraindicated during or within 14 days of MAOI administration. Allow 5 weeks after stopping fluoxetine before starting an MAOI.
- Patients should report symptoms of hyponatremia, including headache, confusion, weakness.
- Side effects: somnolence, insomnia, anxiety, dry mouth, nausea

FLUTICASONE PROPIONATE
(nasal, inhalation)

Brand Names
- Flonase, Flovent

Pharmacologic Class
- Corticosteroid

Mechanism of Action
- Inhibits inflammatory cells (mast cells, eosinophils, basophils, lymphocytes, macrophages, and neutrophils) and release of inflammatory mediators (histamine, eicosanoids, leukotrienes, and cytokines).

Dosage Forms
- Nasal (suspension), inhalation (aerosol, breath-actuated aerosol)

Common Uses
- Treatment of allergic and nonallergic rhinitis, asthma

Quick Facts
- Nasal spray may take several days of regular use for rhinitis symptoms to improve.
- Inhalation dosage forms may take 1 to 2 weeks of regular use for asthma symptoms to improve.
- When using nasal spray, shake gently before each use. Prime before first use and if not used for 7 or more days. Clean nasal applicator and dust cover once per week by running under warm water and air dry.
- When using HFA inhaler, shake gently before use. Prime inhaler before using for the first time, if the canister is dropped, or if it is not used for more than 7 days. Clean inhaler once per week. (Use a cotton swab dampened with water to clean opening where medicine comes out of canister, and wipe inside of mouthpiece with a damp tissue.)
- Patients using inhalation dosage forms should rinse mouth with water, without swallowing, after each use to prevent oral candidiasis.
- Side effects for nasal spray: nasal burning or irritation, epistaxis, headache
- Side effects for inhalation use: upper respiratory tract infection, oropharyngeal pain, sinusitis, headache

FLUTICASONE-SALMETEROL

Brand Names
- Advair Diskus, Advair HFA

Pharmacologic Class
- Combination beta$_2$-agonist and corticosteroid

Mechanism of Action
- Fluticasone inhibits inflammatory cells (mast cells, eosinophils, basophils, lymphocytes, macrophages, and neutrophils) and release of inflammatory mediators (histamine, eicosanoids, leukotrienes, and cytokines). Salmeterol binds to beta$_2$-adrenergic receptors and increases the level of cAMP, which relaxes bronchial smooth muscle.

Dosage Forms
- Inhalation (powder, aerosol liquid)

Common Uses
- Treatment of asthma and COPD

Quick Facts
- When using the Diskus dry powder inhaler, do not exhale into the device, and use only in a level horizontal position. Discard device 1 month after it is removed from the foil pouch.
- When using the HFA inhaler, shake well for 5 seconds before each spray. Prime inhaler before using for the first time, if the canister is dropped, or if it is not used for more than 4 weeks.
- Counsel patients to rinse mouth with water, without swallowing, after each use to prevent oral candidiasis.
- Side effects: upper respiratory tract infection, nasopharynxgitis, oropharyngeal pain, sinusitis, headache

FOLIC ACID

Brand Name
- Folacin-800

Pharmacologic Class
- Vitamin

Mechanism of Action
- Folic acid is converted to tetrahydrofolic acid and methyltetrahydrofolate, which are required for the synthesis of thymidylate, purine nucleotides, and for normal erythropoiesis.

Dosage Forms
- Oral (tablet, capsule), injection solution (IM/IV)

Common Uses
- Treatment of megaloblastic and macrocytic anemias due to folate deficiency

Quick Facts
- Women planning a pregnancy and all women of child-bearing age should take folic acid (0.4 to 0.8 mg/day) to decrease the risk of neural tube defects.
- Doses greater than 0.1 mg/day may obscure pernicious anemia.
- Side effects: bitter or bad taste in mouth, loss of appetite, nausea, confusion, sleep pattern disturbance

FOSINOPRIL

Brand Name
- Monopril

Pharmacologic Class
- ACE inhibitor

Mechanism of Action
- Inhibits the angiotensin converting enzyme (ACE), which prevents the conversion of angiotensin I to angiotensin II, a potent vasoconstrictor.

Dosage Form
- Oral (tablet)

Common Uses
- Treatment of hypertension and heart failure

Quick Facts
- Black Box Warning – Discontinue use as soon as possible if pregnancy is detected.
- Contraindicated in patients with a history of angioedema or concomitant use with aliskiren in diabetic patients.
- Use caution in patients with impaired renal function.
- Patients should avoid potassium supplements or salt substitutes containing potassium without first consulting healthcare provider.
- Take antacids 2 hours before or after medication.
- Side effects: cough, hypotension, dizziness, hyperkalemia, angioedema

FUROSEMIDE

Brand Name
- Lasix

Pharmacologic Class
- Loop diuretic

Mechanism of Action
- Inhibits sodium and chloride reabsorption in proximal and distal tubules, as well as in the ascending loop of Henle.

Dosage Forms
- Oral (tablet, solution), intravenous (solution)

Common Uses
- Treatment of edema associated with heart failure, cirrhosis of the liver or renal disease, acute pulmonary edema, and hypertension

Quick Facts
- Black Box Warning – Furosemide is a potent diuretic which, if given in excessive amounts, can lead to profound diuresis with water and electrolyte depletion.
- Contraindicated in patients with anuria.
- Administer in the morning because of increased diuresis.
- Ototoxicity has been reported with rapid injection, severe renal impairment, higher than recommended doses, hypoproteinemia, or concomitant therapy with aminoglycosides, ethacrynic acid, or other ototoxic drugs.
- Infusion rate should not exceed 4 mg/min.
- Medication can cause electrolyte imbalances including hypokalemia, hyponatremia, hypocalcemia, hypomagnesemia, and hypochloremic alkalosis. Monitor periodically.
- Side effects: hyperuricemia, hyperglycemia, weakness, rash, photosensitivity

GABAPENTIN

Brand Names
- Neurontin, Gralise

Pharmacologic Class
- Anticonvulsant

Mechanism of Action
- Mechanism of action remains unknown. Gabapentin is structurally related to GABA, but it does not interact with GABA receptors or influence the degradation or uptake of GABA.

Dosage Forms
- Oral (tablet, capsule, solution)

Common Uses
- Treatment of postherpetic neuralgia; adjunctive therapy in the treatment of partial seizures (immediate release)

Quick Facts
- Reduce dosage in renal impairment.
- Patients should not use aluminum or magnesium-containing antacids for at least 2 hours before or after taking medication.
- Immediate-release dosage forms can be taken with or without food. Extended-release dosage form should be taken with evening meal.
- Avoid alcohol use.
- Avoid abrupt discontinuation in patients with seizure disorders.
- Side effects: drowsiness, dizziness, nystagmus, ataxia

GEMFIBROZIL

Brand Name
- Lopid

Pharmacologic Class
- Fibric acid derivative

Mechanism of Action
- Activates peroxisome proliferator activated receptor alpha (PPARα) which increases lipolysis, activates lipoprotein lipase, and reduces production of apoprotein C-III. This causes a lowering of VLDL and triglycerides and an increase in HDL.

Dosage Forms
- Oral (tablet, capsule)

Common Uses
- Treatment of hyperlipidemia and hypertriglyceridemia

Quick Facts
- Contraindicated in active liver disease, severe renal disease, and gallbladder disease.
- Concomitant use with statins is contraindicated due to increased risk of myopathy and rhabdomyolysis.
- Patients should report symptoms of cholelithiasis or cholecystitis, which includes right upper abdominal pain, vomiting, fever, and jaundice.
- Administer 30 minutes before morning and evening meals to increase medication absorption.
- Side effects: abdominal pain, dyspepsia, nausea, diarrhea

GLIMEPIRIDE

Brand Name
- Amaryl

Pharmacologic Class
- Sulfonylurea

Mechanism of Action
- Stimulates insulin release from pancreatic beta cells.

Dosage Form
- Oral (tablet)

Common Use
- Treatment of type 2 diabetes

Quick Facts
- Take with breakfast or the first meal of the day.
- Avoid alcohol use.
- Concomitant use with a CYP2C9 inhibitor increases the risk of hypoglycemia.
- Patients should be counseled to monitor for signs of hypoglycemia (sweating, tremor, blurred vision, hunger, headache, etc.) and to always have a source of oral glucose available for treatment.
- Side effects: nausea, dizziness, asthenia, headache

GLIPIZIDE

Brand Name
- Glucotrol

Pharmacologic Class
- Sulfonylurea

Mechanism of Action
- Stimulates insulin release from pancreatic beta cells and may improve insulin sensitivity and decrease hepatic glucose production.

Dosage Form
- Oral (tablet)

Common Use
- Treatment of type 2 diabetes

Quick Facts
- Medication should be taken 30 minutes before a meal, preferably breakfast.
- Avoid alcohol use.
- Concomitant use with a CYP2C9 inhibitor increases the risk of hypoglycemia.
- Patients should be counseled to monitor for signs of hypoglycemia (sweating, tremor, blurred vision, hunger, headache, etc.) and to always have a source of oral glucose available for treatment.
- Side effects: diarrhea, nausea, dyspepsia, headache

GLYBURIDE

Brand Names
- Diabeta, Micronase

Pharmacologic Class
- Sulfonylurea

Mechanism of Action
- Stimulates insulin release from pancreatic beta cells.

Dosage Form
- Oral (tablet)

Common Use
- Treatment of type 2 diabetes

Quick Facts
- Medication has an active metabolite that is renally cleared and may accumulate with renal dysfunction, which can cause prolonged hypoglycemia.
- Take with breakfast or the first meal of the day.
- Avoid alcohol use.
- Patients should be counseled to monitor for signs of hypoglycemia (sweating, tremor, blurred vision, hunger, headache, etc.) and to always have a source of oral glucose available for treatment.
- Side effects: nausea, heartburn, weight gain

GUAIFENESIN-CODEINE

Brand Names
- Robitussin AC, Cheratussin AC, Virtussin AC

Pharmacologic Class
- Combination antitussive and expectorant

Mechanism of Action
- Guaifenesin thins bronchial secretions and increases mucus secretions. Codeine depresses the medullary cough center.

Dosage Forms
- Oral (solution, syrup)

Common Use
- Treatment of cough

Quick Facts
- DEA Schedule V
- Black Box Warning – Respiratory depression and death have occurred in children who received codeine following tonsillectomy and/or adenoidectomy and had evidence of being ultra-rapid metabolizers of codeine due to CYP2D6 polymorphism.
- Contraindications include children younger than 12 years, patients with asthma, and postoperative management in children younger than 18 years following tonsillectomy and/or adenoidectomy.
- Avoid alcohol and other CNS depressants.
- Side effects: constipation, drowsiness, headache, nausea

GUANFACINE

Brand Name
- Intuniv

Pharmacologic Class
- Alpha$_2$-agonist

Mechanism of Action
- Exact mechanism of guanfacine in ADHD is unknown. Stimulates alpha$_2$-adrenergic receptors in the brain, which reduces sympathetic outflow from the CNS to the heart and peripheral vasculature.

Dosage Form
- Oral (tablet)

Common Uses
- Treatment of ADHD and hypertension (immediate release only)

Quick Facts
- Avoid taking with a high-fat meal because it increases absorption.
- Avoid abrupt discontinuation to prevent withdrawal symptoms, which include rebound hypertension, nervousness, and anxiety.
- Dose should be adjusted when used with strong CYP3A4 inhibitors or inducers.
- Patients should avoid becoming dehydrated or over-heated which may potentially increase the risks of hypotension and syncope.
- Side effects: fatigue, bradycardia, hypotension, nausea

HALOPERIDOL

Brand Name
- Haldol

Pharmacologic Class
- Antipsychotic

Mechanism of Action
- Nonselectively blocks postsynaptic dopaminergic D_2 receptors within the mesolimbic and mesocortical systems of the brain.

Dosage Forms
- Oral (tablet, solution), short-acting injection (haloperidol lactate), long-acting injection (haloperidol decanoate)

Common Uses
- Treatment of schizophrenia, hyperactive behavior in children, and Tourette's syndrome

Quick Facts
- Black Box Warning – Elderly patients with dementia-related psychosis treated with antipsychotics are at an increased risk of death compared to placebo. Most deaths appeared to be either cardiovascular (e.g., heart failure, sudden death) or infectious (e.g., pneumonia) in nature.
- Can prolong the QT interval.
- Patients should be counseled to report signs of extrapyramidal symptoms, tardive dyskinesia (restlessness, tremor, stiffness, etc.) or neuroleptic malignant syndrome (sweating, fever, muscle rigidity, etc.).
- Side effects: hypotension, dry mouth, blurred vision, constipation

HYDRALAZINE

Brand Name
- Apresoline

Pharmacologic Class
- Vasodilator

Mechanism of Action
- Exact mechanism of action is unknown, but is theorized to interfere with calcium movement in vascular smooth muscle. Hydralazine directly relaxes arteriole smooth muscle with little effect on venous smooth muscle.

Dosage Forms
- Oral (tablet), injection solution (IM/IV)

Common Use
- Treatment of hypertension

Quick Facts
- Medication may cause drug-induced lupus erythematosus (DILE), serum sickness, hemolytic anemia, vasculitis, and glomerulonephritis. Symptoms of DILE include fever, joint and muscle aches, and fatigue.
- A complete blood count (CBC) and an antinuclear antibody (ANA) titer determination should be performed before and periodically during prolonged therapy.
- Peripheral neuropathy has been reported. If this occurs, pyridoxine should be added to the patient's regimen.
- Administration with food increases bioavailability. Administer consistently with regard to meals.
- Side effects: headache, palpitations, tachycardia, angina pectoris

HYDROCHLOROTHIAZIDE

Brand Names
- Microzide, HydroDiuril

Pharmacologic Class
- Thiazide diuretic

Mechanism of Action
- Inhibits sodium and chloride reabsorption in the renal distal convoluted tubule.

Dosage Forms
- Oral (tablet, capsule)

Common Uses
- Treatment of hypertension and edema

Quick Facts
- Contraindicated in patients with anuria or who have a hypersensitivity to sulfonamides.
- Administer in the morning to prevent nocturia.
- Medication can cause electrolyte imbalances including hypokalemia, hyponatremia, hypercalcemia, and hypomagnesemia. Monitor periodically.
- Use with caution in patients with gout. Medication can cause hyperuricemia.
- Use with caution in patients with diabetes. Medication can cause hyperglycemia.
- Usually ineffective in patients with a CrCl < 30 mL/min.
- Side effects: orthostatic hypotension, dizziness, weakness, photosensitivity, rash

HYDROCODONE-ACETAMINOPHEN

Brand Names
- Norco, Vicodin, Lortab

Pharmacologic Class
- Opioid analgesic combination

Mechanism of Action
- Hydrocodone binds to the mu opioid receptor, which reduces neuronal cell excitability and transmission of nociceptive impulses. Acetaminophen inhibits prostaglandin synthesis in the CNS and blocks pain impulse generation peripherally.

Dosage Forms
- Oral (tablet, solution)

Common Use
- Treatment of moderate to severe pain

Quick Facts
- DEA Schedule II
- Black Box Warnings – Serious, life-threatening, or fatal respiratory depression may occur. Concomitant use with benzodiazepines increases risk of sedation, respiratory depression, coma, or death. Concomitant use with CYP3A4 inhibitors, or discontinuation of CYP3A4 inducers, can result in a fatal overdose of hydrocodone-acetaminophen. Prolonged use of hydrocodone-acetaminophen during pregnancy can result in neonatal opioid withdrawal syndrome. Acetaminophen has been associated with cases of acute liver failure.
- Patients should not exceed more than 4 grams of acetaminophen in a 24-hour period.
- Side effects: drowsiness, constipation, dizziness, nausea, vomiting

HYDROCORTISONE (topical)

Brand Names
- Westcort, Locoid

Pharmacologic Class
- Corticosteroid

Mechanism of Action
- Hydrocortisone has anti-inflammatory, antipruritic, and vasoconstrictive properties. The anti-inflammatory effect is believed to be due to stimulation of phospholipase A_2 inhibitory proteins. These proteins subsequently block the release of arachidonic acid, which is a precursor to leukotrienes and prostaglandins.

Dosage Forms
- Topical (cream, lotion, ointment, gel, solution)

Common Uses
- Treatment of inflammatory and pruritic manifestations of corticosteroid-responsive dermatoses

Quick Facts
- Contact prescriber if no improvement is seen within 2 weeks.
- Topical steroid overuse can cause thinning of the skin and striae.
- Do not use with bandages, wraps, or other occlusive dressings unless directed by prescriber.
- Apply sparingly and wash hands after application.
- Side effects: pruritis, burning sensation, hypothalamic-pituitary-adrenal axis suppression

HYDROMORPHONE

Brand Names
- Dilaudid, Exalgo

Pharmacologic Class
- Opioid analgesic

Mechanism of Action
- Binds to the mu opioid receptor, which reduces neuronal cell excitability and transmission of nociceptive impulses.

Dosage Forms
- Oral (tablet, solution), injection solution (IM/IV/SubQ), rectal (suppository)

Common Use
- Treatment of moderate to severe pain

Quick Facts
- DEA Schedule II
- Black Box Warnings – Serious, life-threatening, or fatal respiratory depression may occur. Concomitant use with benzodiazepines increases risk of sedation, respiratory depression, coma, or death. Prolonged use of hydromorphone during pregnancy can result in neonatal opioid withdrawal syndrome.
- MAOIs can potentiate the effects of hydromorphone. Avoid concomitant use of MAOIs or within 14 days of MAOI discontinuation.
- Concomitant use with serotonergic drugs may cause serotonin syndrome.
- Avoid abrupt discontinuation to prevent withdrawal symptoms.
- Side effects: somnolence, constipation, pruritis, sweating, dry mouth

HYDROXYCHLOROQUINE

Brand Name
- Plaquenil

Pharmacologic Class
- Antimalarial

Mechanism of Action
- Mechanism of action remains unknown. In malaria, hydroxychloroquine may increase the pH of certain components in sensitive parasites and interfere with lysosomal degradation of hemoglobin. As an antirheumatic, hydroxychloroquine is thought to act as an immunosuppressant by inhibiting the production of rheumatoid factor and acute phase reactants.

Dosage Form
- Oral (tablet)

Common Uses
- Treatment of rheumatoid arthritis, discoid and systemic lupus erythematosus, and malaria

Quick Facts
- Take with food or milk to decrease GI upset.
- Can cause QT prolongation.
- Monitoring parameters include CBC, renal function tests, and LFTs at baseline and periodically thereafter. Obtain ophthalmologic exam at baseline and annually after 5 years of use.
- Side effects: visual disturbances, blood dyscrasias, irritability, abnormal skin pigmentation, ataxia

HYDROXYZINE

Brand Names
- Atarax (hydroxyzine hydrochloride), Vistaril (hydroxyzine pamoate)

Pharmacologic Class
- H_1 antagonist

Mechanism of Action
- Antagonist at peripheral H_1 receptors. Also suppresses histamine activity in the subcortical region of the CNS.

Dosage Forms
- Hydroxyzine hydrochloride: oral (tablet, syrup), intramuscular (solution)
- Hydroxyzine pamoate: oral (capsule)

Common Uses
- Treatment of anxiety, pruritis, nausea, and vomiting (intramuscular dosage form)

Quick Facts
- Use with caution in patients with asthma, BPH, and glaucoma.
- Avoid alcohol and other CNS depressants while taking medication.
- May prolong the QT interval.
- Side effects: drowsiness, dry mouth, headache

HYOSCYAMINE

Brand Names
- Levbid, Levsin

Pharmacologic Class
- Anticholinergic

Mechanism of Action
- Blocks the action of acetylcholine at parasympathetic sties in smooth muscle, secretory gland tissue, and in the CNS.

Dosage Forms
- Oral (tablet, sublingual tablet, disintegrating tablet, solution), injection solution (IM/IV/SubQ)

Common Use
- Treatment of irritable bowel syndrome

Quick Facts
- Contraindications include GI or urinary tract obstruction, glaucoma, myasthenia gravis, and severe ulcerative colitis.
- Do not take with antacids, as they may decrease the absorption of hyoscyamine.
- Use with caution in patients with renal impairment.
- Medication can cause anhidrosis, therefore use caution during hot weather and with activities leading to an increase in core temperature or dehydration.
- Side effects: dry mouth, constipation, urinary retention, blurred vision, tachycardia

IBANDRONATE

Brand Name
- Boniva

Pharmacologic Class
- Bisphosphonate

Mechanism of Action
- Inhibits osteoclast-mediated bone resorption.

Dosage Forms
- Oral (tablet), intravenous (solution)

Common Uses
- Treatment and prevention of postmenopausal osteoporosis

Quick Facts
- Medication should be taken in the morning at least 60 minutes before the first food, beverage, and other medications of the day with 6 to 8 oz. of plain water. Patient should stay upright for at least 60 minutes and until after eating to prevent esophageal irritation.
- Products containing calcium, magnesium, or aluminum should be taken at a separate time.
- Side effects: abdominal pain, acid regurgitation, constipation, diarrhea, esophagitis
- Less common side effects: osteonecrosis of the jaw, atypical femur fracture

IBUPROFEN

Brand Names
- Motrin, Advil

Pharmacologic Class
- NSAID

Mechanism of Action
- Prevents the synthesis of prostaglandins by inhibiting the cyclooxygenase-1 and cyclooxygenase-2 (COX-1 and 2) enzymes.

Dosage Forms
- Oral (tablet, chewable tablet, capsule, suspension), intravenous (solution)

Common Uses
- Treatment of mild to moderate pain, rheumatoid arthritis, osteoarthritis, and juvenile arthritis

Quick Facts
- Black Box Warnings – Increased risk of cardiovascular thrombotic events and GI bleeding, ulceration, and perforation. Contraindicated in the setting of coronary artery bypass graft surgery.
- Contraindicated in patients with a history of asthma, urticaria, or other allergic-type reactions after taking aspirin or other NSAIDs.
- Pregnant patients should avoid use starting in the third trimester due to the risk of premature closure of the ductus arteriosus.
- Use with caution in patients with renal or hepatic impairment.
- Side effects: heartburn, nausea, edema, diarrhea, abdominal pain

IMIQUIMOD

Brand Names
- Aldara, Zyclara

Pharmacologic Class
- Immune modulator

Mechanism of Action
- Mechanism of action remains unknown. Appears to act as a Toll-like receptor 7 agonist, which leads to increased markers for cytokines and immune cells.

Dosage Form
- Topical (cream)

Common Uses
- Treatment of external genital warts, superficial basal cell carcinoma, and actinic keratosis

Quick Facts
- Wash hands before and after application.
- Apply a thin film to treatment area and rub in until the cream is no longer visible.
- For most indications, cream should be left on the skin for approximately 8 hours, then removed by washing with soap and water.
- Do not use occlusive dressings over treated areas.
- Medication can cause hypopigmentation or hyperpigmentation of treated areas, which may be permanent.
- Side effects: itching, burning, vesicles, weeping, dryness of skin

INDOMETHACIN

Brand Names
- Indocin, Tivorbex

Pharmacologic Class
- NSAID

Mechanism of Action
- Prevents the synthesis of prostaglandins by inhibiting the cyclooxygenase-1 and cyclooxygenase-2 (COX-1 and 2) enzymes.

Dosage Forms
- Oral (capsule, suspension), intravenous (powder for solution), rectal (suppository)

Common Uses
- Treatment of mild to moderate pain, rheumatoid arthritis, osteoarthritis, gout, and ankylosing spondylitis

Quick Facts
- Black Box Warnings – Increased risk of cardiovascular thrombotic events and GI bleeding, ulceration, and perforation. Contraindicated in the setting of coronary artery bypass graft surgery.
- Contraindicated in patients with a history of asthma, urticaria, or other allergic-type reactions after taking aspirin or other NSAIDs.
- Pregnant patients should avoid use starting at 30 weeks gestation due to the risk of premature closure of the ductus arteriosus.
- Use with caution in patients with renal or hepatic impairment.
- Side effects: dyspepsia, nausea, vomiting, headache, diarrhea, constipation, abdominal pain

INSULIN ASPART

Brand Names
- Novolog, Fiasp

Pharmacologic Class
- Insulin, rapid-acting

Mechanism of Action
- Binds to the insulin receptors on muscle and fat cells and lowers blood glucose by increasing the cellular uptake of glucose and simultaneously inhibiting the output of glucose from the liver.

Dosage Form
- Subcutaneous (solution)

Common Uses
- Treatment of type 1 and type 2 diabetes

Quick Facts
- Novolog should be administered 5 to 10 minutes before a meal. Fiasp should be administered at the start of a meal or 20 minutes after starting a meal.
- Refrigerate unused vials, pens, and cartridges. Used vials and pens can be stored in refrigerator or at room temperature and should be discarded 28 days after initial use. Used cartridges should be stored at room temperature and discarded after 28 days.
- Rotate injection sites to prevent inflammation and lipodystrophy.
- Side effects: hypoglycemia, lipodystrophy, rash

INSULIN DETEMIR

Brand Name
- Levemir

Pharmacologic Class
- Insulin, long-acting

Mechanism of Action
- Binds to the insulin receptors on muscle and fat cells and lowers blood glucose by increasing the cellular uptake of glucose and simultaneously inhibiting the output of glucose from the liver.

Dosage Form
- Subcutaneous (solution)

Common Uses
- Treatment of type 1 and type 2 diabetes

Quick Facts
- Administer once daily or in divided doses twice daily. Once daily administration should be given with the evening meal or at bedtime.
- Refrigerate unused vials and pens. If refrigeration is not possible, vials and pens can be stored at room temperature, then discarded 42 days after it was first kept out of refrigerator even if the vial or pen still contains insulin. Used vials and pens can be stored in refrigerator or at room temperature and should be discarded 42 days after initial use.
- Do not dilute or mix with any other insulin or solution.
- Rotate injection sites to prevent inflammation and lipodystrophy.
- Side effects: hypoglycemia, lipodystrophy, rash

INSULIN GLARGINE

Brand Names
- Lantus, Toujeo, Basaglar

Pharmacologic Class
- Insulin, long-acting

Mechanism of Action
- Binds to the insulin receptors on muscle and fat cells and lowers blood glucose by increasing the cellular uptake of glucose and simultaneously inhibiting the output of glucose from the liver.

Dosage Form
- Subcutaneous (solution)

Common Uses
- Treatment of type 1 and type 2 diabetes

Quick Facts
- Administer once daily at the same time every day.
- Unopened vials and pens of Lantus can be stored at room temperature for 28 days or in refrigerator until expiration date. In-use vials can be stored at room temperature or refrigerated for up to 28 days. In-use pens should be stored at room temperature for up to 28 days.
- Unopened pens of Basaglar can be stored at room temperature for 28 days or in refrigerator until expiration date. In-use pens should be stored at room temperature for up to 28 days.
- Unopened pens of Toujeo should be stored in refrigerator, and in-use pens should be stored at room temperature for up to 28 days.
- Do not dilute or mix with any other insulin or solution.
- Rotate injection sites to prevent inflammation and lipodystrophy.
- Side effects: hypoglycemia, lipodystrophy, rash

INSULIN LISPRO

Brand Names
- Humalog, Admelog

Pharmacologic Class
- Insulin, rapid-acting

Mechanism of Action
- Binds to the insulin receptors on muscle and fat cells and lowers blood glucose by increasing the cellular uptake of glucose and simultaneously inhibiting the output of glucose from the liver.

Dosage Form
- Subcutaneous (solution)

Common Uses
- Treatment of type 1 and type 2 diabetes

Quick Facts
- Administer within 15 minutes before or immediately after a meal.
- Unopened vials and pens can be stored at room temperature for 28 days or in refrigerator until expiration date. In-use vials can be stored at room temperature or refrigerated for up to 28 days. In-use pens should be stored at room temperature for up to 28 days.
- Rotate injection sites to prevent inflammation and lipodystrophy.
- Side effects: hypoglycemia, lipodystrophy, rash

INSULIN, REGULAR HUMAN

Brand Names
- Novolin R, Humulin R

Pharmacologic Class
- Insulin, rapid-acting

Mechanism of Action
- Binds to the insulin receptors on muscle and fat cells and lowers blood glucose by increasing the cellular uptake of glucose and simultaneously inhibiting the output of glucose from the liver.

Dosage Forms
- Subcutaneous (solution), intravenous (solution)

Common Uses
- Treatment of type 1 and type 2 diabetes

Quick Facts
- Administer 30 minutes prior to a meal.
- Store unused vials of Humulin R in refrigerator. In-use vials can be stored at room temperature for 31 days.
- Unused vials of Novolin R can be stored at room temperature for up to 42 days or in refrigerator until expiration date. In-use vials can be stored at room temperature for up to 42 days.
- Rotate injection sites to prevent inflammation and lipodystrophy.
- Side effects: hypoglycemia, lipodystrophy, rash

IPRATROPIUM

Brand Name
- Atrovent

Pharmacologic Class
- Anticholinergic

Mechanism of Action
- Blocks the action of acetylcholine at parasympathetic sites in bronchial smooth muscle causing bronchodilation. When applied locally to nasal mucosa, ipratropium inhibits serous and seromucous gland secretions.

Dosage Forms
- Inhalation (aerosol, solution), nasal (solution)

Common Uses
- Treatment of COPD through inhalation dosage forms and rhinorrhea associated with the common cold or seasonal allergic rhinitis through nasal dosage forms

Quick Facts
- Avoid spraying in or near eyes as this may cause eye pain, temporary blurring of vision, visual halos, mydriasis, or new onset or worsening of narrow-angle glaucoma.
- Use with caution in patients with narrow-angle glaucoma, BPH, or bladder neck obstruction.
- HFA inhaler should be primed prior to first use or if not used in more than 3 days by spraying 2 times. Mouthpiece should be cleaned at least once per week by removing the canister and running under warm water, then air-drying completely.
- Nasal spray should be primed prior to first use or if not used in more than 7 days by spraying 7 times. If not used in more than 24 hours, prime by spraying 2 times.
- Side effects from the nasal spray: headache, nasal burning, coughing, upper respiratory tract infection
- Side effects from inhalation use: headache, upper respiratory tract infection, dizziness, dry mouth

IRBESARTAN

Brand Name
- Avapro

Pharmacologic Class
- ARB

Mechanism of Action
- Blocks the binding of angiotensin II to the angiotensin II type-1 receptor on vascular smooth muscle, which prevents vasoconstriction and the secretion of aldosterone.

Dosage Form
- Oral (tablet)

Common Uses
- Treatment of hypertension and diabetic nephropathy

Quick Facts
- Black Box Warning – Discontinue use as soon as possible if pregnancy is detected.
- Contraindicated with concomitant use with aliskiren in diabetic patients.
- NSAIDs may reduce antihypertensive effect and increase the risk of renal dysfunction.
- Patients should avoid potassium supplements or salt substitutes containing potassium without first consulting healthcare provider.
- Side effects: fatigue, dyspepsia, diarrhea, dizziness

ISOSORBIDE MONONITRATE

Brand Name
- Imdur

Pharmacologic Class
- Antianginal/Vasodilator

Mechanism of Action
- Acts as a prodrug for nitric oxide, which relaxes vascular smooth muscle and causes dilation of peripheral veins and arteries, with more prominent effects on veins to decrease cardiac preload.

Dosage Form
- Oral (tablet)

Common Uses
- Prevention and treatment of angina pectoris caused by coronary artery disease

Quick Facts
- Medication should not be used to treat acute anginal attacks because onset of action is not rapid enough.
- Immediate-release tablet should be administered twice daily with doses 7 hours apart to prevent tolerance. Extended-release tablets should be taken in the morning with half a glass of liquid. Extended-release tablets may be divided in half.
- Avoid concomitant use with PDE-5 inhibitors due to the risk of severe hypotension, syncope, or myocardial ischemia.
- Side effects: headache, dizziness, lightheadedness, flushing

KETOCONAZOLE

Brand Names
- Nizoral, Ketodan, Extina, Xolegel

Pharmacologic Class
- Antifungal

Mechanism of Action
- Decreases the synthesis of ergosterol, which is an essential component of fungal cell membranes.

Dosage Forms
- Oral (tablet), topical (cream, foam, gel, shampoo)

Common Uses
- Treatment of systemic fungal infections (oral dosage form), tinea corporis, tinea cruris, tinea pedis, seborrheic dermatitis, and dandruff (topical dosage forms)

Quick Facts
- Black Box Warnings – Oral ketoconazole should only be used when other antifungal therapies are unavailable or not tolerated and the potential benefits outweigh the risks. Serious hepatoxicity, including cases with a fatal outcome or requiring liver transplantation has occurred. Concomitant use with cisapride, disopyramide, dofetilide, dronedarone, methadone, pimozide, quinidine, and ranolazine is contraindicated due to the possible occurrence of ventricular arrhythmias such as torsades de pointes.
- Potent inhibitor of CYP3A4.
- Absorption is pH-dependent. Avoid using with antacids, H_2RAs, and PPIs.
- Side effects with oral use: nausea, vomiting
- Side effects with topical use: pruritis and application site reaction. Shampoo can cause oiliness and dryness of the hair and scalp and altered hair texture.

LABETALOL

Brand Names
▪ Normodyne, Trandate

Pharmacologic Class
▪ $Beta_1/beta_2$-blocker and $alpha_1$-blocker

Mechanism of Action
▪ Blocks stimulation of $beta_1$ (myocardial) and $beta_2$ (pulmonary, vascular)-adrenergic receptors which reduces cardiac output, reduces exercise-induced tachycardia and/or isoproterenol-induced tachycardia, and reduces reflex orthostatic tachycardia. Blockade of $alpha_1$-adrenergic receptors causes vasodilation of blood vessels.

Dosage Forms
▪ Oral (tablet), intravenous (solution)

Common Use
▪ Treatment of hypertension

Quick Facts
▪ Contraindications include bronchial asthma or related bronchial spastic condition, 2nd or 3rd degree AV block, cardiogenic shock, severe bradycardia, and conditions associated with severe and prolonged hypotension.
▪ Often used to treat chronic hypertension in pregnancy.
▪ Avoid abrupt discontinuation.
▪ Use with caution in patients with hepatic impairment.
▪ Can be taken with or without food but must be consistent.
▪ Side effects: hypotension, dizziness, fatigue, nausea

LAMOTRIGINE

Brand Name
- Lamictal

Pharmacologic Class
- Anticonvulsant

Mechanism of Action
- Mechanism of action remains unknown. Lamotrigine may produce its anticonvulsant effect by blocking voltage-sensitive sodium channels, which stabilizes neuronal membranes and modulates presynaptic release of excitatory amino acids, glutamate, and aspartate.

Dosage Forms
- Oral (tablet, chewable tablet, disintegrating tablet)

Common Uses
- Treatment of epilepsy (partial seizures, generalized seizures of Lennox-Gastaut syndrome, primary generalized tonic-clonic seizures) and bipolar disorder

Quick Facts
- Black Box Warning – Life-threatening skin reactions including Stevens-Johnson syndrome and toxic epidermal necrolysis have occurred. Incidence is higher in pediatric patients than adults. Risk may be increased when coadministered with valproic acid, high starting doses, or rapid increases in dose.
- Valproic acid increases lamotrigine concentrations by more than two-fold. Estrogen-containing oral contraceptives decrease lamotrigine concentrations by approximately 50%.
- Patients should immediately report symptoms of aseptic meningitis, including headache, stiff neck, fever, nausea, and vomiting.
- Side effects: dizziness, headache, diplopia, ataxia

LANSOPRAZOLE

Brand Name
- Prevacid

Pharmacologic Class
- PPI

Mechanism of Action
- Suppresses gastric acid secretion by inhibiting the H^+/K^+-ATPase pump in parietal cells, blocking the final step of acid production.

Dosage Forms
- Oral (disintegrating tablet, capsule)

Common Uses
- Treatment of GERD, erosive esophagitis, Zollinger-Ellison syndrome, and *H. pylori* eradication; prevention of NSAID-associated gastric ulcers

Quick Facts
- Take at least 30 to 60 minutes before eating.
- Do not abruptly discontinue. Medication should be tapered to avoid acid rebound.
- Use with caution with other medications that require an acidic pH for absorption, including itraconazole, ketoconazole, iron, etc.
- Patients taking long term should have adequate calcium and vitamin D intake. (Calcium citrate formulations will have improved absorption in basic pH).
- Short-term side effects: headache, abdominal pain, diarrhea, constipation
- Long-term side effects: increased risk of osteoporosis or fracture, vitamin B_{12} deficiency, hypomagnesemia

LATANOPROST

Brand Names
- Xalatan, Xelpros

Pharmacologic Class
- Prostaglandin analog

Mechanism of Action
- Decreases intraocular pressure by increasing the outflow of aqueous humor through the trabecular meshwork and uveoscleral pathway.

Dosage Forms
- Ophthalmic (solution, emulsion)

Common Uses
- Treatment of open-angle glaucoma and ocular hypertension

Quick Facts
- Remove contact lenses before instilling medication and allow at least 15 minutes before reinserting.
- Wait at least 5 minutes before administering other ophthalmic products.
- Store unopened bottle in refrigerator. Once opened, can be stored at room temperature for 6 weeks.
- Side effects: pigment changes to eyelids and eyelashes, increased brown pigmentation of the iris, growth of eyelashes, conjunctival hyperemia, ocular pruritis

LETROZOLE

Brand Name
- Femara

Pharmacologic Class
- Aromatase inhibitor

Mechanism of Action
- Non-steroidal aromatase inhibitor that blocks the conversion of androgens to estrogens in peripheral tissues.

Dosage Form
- Oral (tablet)

Common Use
- Treatment of breast cancer in postmenopausal women

Quick Facts
- Can decrease bone mineral density. (Monitor at baseline and every 1 to 2 years with DEXA scan.)
- Consider monitoring total cholesterol and LDL during therapy.
- Medication should not be used for the treatment of breast cancer in premenopausal women.
- Side effects: hot flashes, fatigue, rash, vomiting, nausea

LEVALBUTEROL

Brand Name
- Xopenex

Pharmacologic Class
- Beta$_2$-agonist

Mechanism of Action
- Relaxes bronchial smooth muscle by binding to beta$_2$-adrenergic receptors.

Dosage Forms
- Inhalation (aerosol, aerosol powder, solution)

Common Use
- Treatment of asthma

Quick Facts
- HFA inhaler should be shaken well before use, and primed prior to first use and when inhaler has not been used for more than 3 days by spraying into air 3 to 4 times.
- Mouthpiece of HFA inhaler should be cleaned at least once per week by removing the canister and running under warm water, then air-drying completely.
- Side effects: palpitations, tremors, dizziness, cough, nervousness

LEVETIRACETAM

Brand Names
- Keppra, Elepsia XR, Roweepra, Spritam

Pharmacologic Class
- Anticonvulsant

Mechanism of Action
- Mechanism of action remains unknown. Anticonvulsant effect may be due to modulation of synaptic neurotransmitter release through binding to the synaptic vesicle protein SV2A in the brain.

Dosage Forms
- Oral (tablet, solution, tablet for suspension), intravenous (solution)

Common Use
- Treatment of epilepsy (adjunct therapy for partial seizure, tonic-clonic seizure, myoclonic seizure)

Quick Facts
- Patients should report new or worsening depression, suicidal thoughts or behavior, or unusual changes in mood or behavior.
- Use with caution in patients with renal impairment.
- Avoid abrupt discontinuation, as this may increase seizure frequency.
- Side effects: somnolence, dizziness, asthenia, infection

LEVOCETIRIZINE

Brand Name
- Xyzal

Pharmacologic Class
- H_1 antagonist

Mechanism of Action
- Competitively inhibits histamine at H_1 receptor sites.

Dosage Forms
- Oral (tablet, solution)

Common Uses
- Treatment of seasonal and perennial allergic rhinitis, chronic idiopathic urticaria

Quick Facts
- Administer in the evening with or without food.
- Use with caution in patients with mild to severe renal impairment. Use is contraindicated in end-stage renal disease (CrCl < 10 mL/min).
- Avoid alcohol and other CNS depressants while taking medication.
- Side effects in patients age 12 and older: somnolence, nasopharyngitis, dry mouth, pharyngitis
- Side effects in children under age 12: somnolence, pyrexia, cough, epistaxis

LEVOFLOXACIN (systemic)

Brand Name
- Levaquin

Pharmacologic Class
- Fluoroquinolone antibiotic

Mechanism of Action
- Prevents the synthesis of bacterial DNA by inhibiting DNA gyrase (topoisomerase II) and topoisomerase IV.

Dosage Forms
- Oral (tablet, solution), intravenous (solution)

Common Uses
- Treatment of hospital or community-acquired pneumonia, UTIs, skin and skin structure infections, sinusitis, and acute exacerbation of chronic bronchitis

Quick Facts
- Black Box Warnings – Risk of tendinitis, tendon rupture, peripheral neuropathy, CNS effects, and exacerbation of myasthenia gravis.
- Take medication 2 hours before or 2 hours after aluminum or magnesium-containing antacids or products containing calcium, iron, or zinc.
- May cause QT prolongation.
- Diabetic patients should carefully monitor blood glucose.
- Drink plenty of fluids to prevent crystalluria.
- Side effects: nausea, rash, diarrhea, sun sensitivity

LEVOTHYROXINE

Brand Names
- Synthroid, Levoxyl, Levothroid, Tirosint, Unithroid

Pharmacologic Class
- Thyroid product

Mechanism of Action
- Levothyroxine is a synthetic form of thyroxine (T_4). T_4 is converted to its active metabolite, L-triiodothyronine (T_3). T_4 and T_3 exert their physiological actions through control of DNA transcription and protein synthesis. This results in an increased metabolic rate, decreased TSH production by the pituitary gland, and effects on lipid and carbohydrate metabolism.

Dosage Forms
- Oral (tablet, capsule, solution), intravenous (solution)

Common Uses
- Treatment of hypothyroidism, pituitary TSH suppression, and myxedema coma (injectable form)

Quick Facts
- Black Box Warning – Medication should not be used for the treatment of obesity or for weight loss. High doses may produce serious or life-threatening toxic effects.
- Administer in the morning, preferably on an empty stomach, 30 to 60 minutes before breakfast.
- Do not administer within 4 hours of calcium or iron-containing products or bile acid sequestrants.
- Pregnancy may require higher doses.
- Side effects if dose is too high: palpitations, sweating, weight loss

LIDOCAINE (topical patch)

Brand Name
- Lidoderm

Pharmacologic Class
- Topical anesthetic

Mechanism of Action
- Produces local anesthesia by blocking sodium ion channels required for the initiation and conduction of nerve impulses.

Dosage Form
- Topical (patch)

Common Use
- Treatment of pain associated with postherpetic neuralgia

Quick Facts
- Use with caution in patients receiving Class I anti-arrhythmic medications due to potentially synergistic effects.
- Apply the prescribed number of patches (maximum of 3) for a maximum of 12 hours within a 24-hour period. Patches may be cut.
- Do not apply patches to broken or inflamed skin.
- Avoid showering, swimming, or bathing while wearing patch, and do not apply external heat to application site.
- Side effects: blisters, bruising, discoloration, edema, pruritis, and irritation, which usually resolves within a few minutes to hours

LINACLOTIDE

Brand Name
- Linzess

Pharmacologic Class
- Guanylate cyclase-C agonist

Mechanism of Action
- Linaclotide and its active metabolite bind to guanylate cyclase-C (GC-C) on the luminal surface of intestinal epithelium. This increases intra- and extracellular levels of cGMP, which stimulates the secretion of chloride and bicarbonate into the intestinal lumen, resulting in increased intestinal fluid and accelerated transit.

Dosage Form
- Oral (capsule)

Common Uses
- Treatment of irritable bowel syndrome with constipation and chronic idiopathic constipation

Quick Facts
- Black Box Warning – Risk of serious dehydration in pediatric patients. Contraindicated in patients < 6 years of age. Avoid use in patients 6 years to less than 18 years of age. The safety and effectiveness of linaclotide has not been established in patients less than 18 years of age.
- Contraindicated in patients with known or suspected mechanical GI obstruction.
- Administer on an empty stomach at least 30 minutes prior to the first meal of the day.
- Patients should be counseled to report symptoms of severe diarrhea or abdominal pain.
- Side effects: diarrhea, abdominal pain, flatulence, abdominal distension

LINAGLIPTAN

Brand Name
- Tradjenta

Pharmacologic Class
- DPP-4 inhibitor

Mechanism of Action
- Prevents the dipeptidyl peptidase-4 (DPP-4) enzyme from degrading the incretin hormones glucagon-like peptide-1 (GLP-1) and glucose-dependent insulinotropic polypeptide (GIP). These hormones increase insulin release and decrease glucagon levels.

Dosage Form
- Oral (tablet)

Common Use
- Treatment of type 2 diabetes

Quick Facts
- Patients should be counseled to report symptoms of congestive heart failure, acute pancreatitis, and bullous pemphigoid.
- Medication is a CYP3A4 and P-glycoprotein substrate, and levels will be decreased when used concomitantly with strong inducers, including rifampin, phenytoin, etc.
- Side effects: nasopharyngitis, hypoglycemia, arthralgia

LIRAGLUTIDE

Brand Names
- Victoza, Saxenda

Pharmacologic Class
- GLP-1 receptor agonist

Mechanism of Action
- Analog of incretin (glucagon-like peptide 1), which increases insulin secretion, decreases glucagon secretion, slows gastric emptying, and decreases food intake.

Dosage Form
- Subcutaneous (solution)

Common Use
- Treatment of type 2 diabetes

Quick Facts
- Black Box Warning – Causes an increased incidence of thyroid C-cell tumors in rats. The human relevance has not been determined. Exenatide extended-release is contraindicated in patients with a personal or family history of medullary thyroid carcinoma or in patients with Multiple Endocrine Neoplasia syndrome type 2 (MEN 2).
- Refrigerate unused pens. Used pens can be stored in refrigerator or at room temperature and should be discarded 30 days after initial use.
- Administer once daily without regard to meals.
- May cause pancreatitis.
- Side effects: nausea, vomiting, diarrhea, headache

LISDEXAMFETAMINE

Brand Name
- Vyvanse

Pharmacologic Class
- CNS stimulant

Mechanism of Action
- Exact mechanism of lisdexamfetamine in ADHD and binge eating disorder is unknown. Lisdexamfetamine is a prodrug of dextroamphetamine, which blocks the reuptake of norepinephrine and dopamine in presynaptic nerve endings and increases their release into the extraneuronal space.

Dosage Forms
- Oral (capsule, chewable tablet)

Common Uses
- Treatment of ADHD and binge eating disorder

Quick Facts
- DEA Schedule II
- Black Box Warning – High potential for abuse, and administration for prolonged periods of time may lead to dependence. Misuse may cause sudden death and serious cardiovascular adverse reactions.
- Use is contraindicated during or within 14 days of MAOI administration, including linezolid or methylene blue.
- Gradually increase dosing and avoid abrupt discontinuation to prevent withdrawal symptoms.
- Side effects: loss of appetite, weight loss, dry mouth, nausea, diarrhea, anxiety

LISINOPRIL

Brand Names
- Prinivil, Zestril, Qbrelis

Pharmacologic Class
- ACE inhibitor

Mechanism of Action
- Inhibits the angiotensin converting enzyme (ACE), which prevents the conversion of angiotensin I to angiotensin II, a potent vasoconstrictor.

Dosage Forms
- Oral (tablet, solution)

Common Uses
- Treatment of hypertension, heart failure, and acute MI

Quick Facts
- Black Box Warning – Discontinue use as soon as possible if pregnancy is detected
- Contraindicated in patients with a history of angioedema, concomitant use with aliskiren in diabetic patients, concomitant use with neprilysin inhibitor, or within 36 hours of switching to or from a neprilysin inhibitor.
- Use caution in patients with impaired renal function.
- Patients should avoid potassium supplements or salt substitutes containing potassium without first consulting healthcare provider.
- Side effects: cough, dizziness, headache, hyperkalemia, fatigue

LISINOPRIL-HYDROCHLOROTHIAZIDE

Brand Names
- Prinzide, Zestoretic

Pharmacologic Class
- Combination ACE inhibitor and thiazide diuretic

Mechanism of Action
- Lisinopril inhibits the angiotensin converting enzyme (ACE), which prevents the conversion of angiotensin I to angiotensin II, a potent vasoconstrictor. Hydrochlorothiazide inhibits sodium and chloride reabsorption in the renal distal convoluted tubule.

Dosage Form
- Oral (tablet)

Common Use
- Treatment of hypertension

Quick Facts
- Black Box Warning – Discontinue use as soon as possible if pregnancy is detected.
- Contraindicated in patients with anuria, hypersensitivity to sulfonamides, a history of angioedema, concomitant use with aliskiren in diabetic patients, concomitant use with neprilysin inhibitor, or within 36 hours of switching to or from a neprilysin inhibitor.
- Patients should avoid potassium supplements or salt substitutes containing potassium without first consulting healthcare provider.
- Side effects: cough, dizziness, headache, orthostatic hypotension, fatigue

LITHIUM CARBONATE

Brand Names
- Lithobid, Eskalith

Pharmacologic Class
- Antimanic

Mechanism of Action
- Mechanism of action is unknown. Its mood-stabilizing effects may be due to a decrease in the release of excitatory neurotransmitters (dopamine and glutamate) and an increase in inhibitory neurotransmission (GABA). Lithium also targets secondary-messenger systems (adenyl cyclase, phosphoinositide pathways, and protein kinase C), which may decrease excitatory neurotransmission.

Dosage Forms
- Oral (tablet, capsule)

Common Use
- Treatment of bipolar disorder

Quick Facts
- Black Box Warning – Lithium toxicity is closely related to serum lithium levels and can occur at doses close to therapeutic levels. Facilities for prompt and accurate serum lithium determinations should be available before initiating therapy.
- Patients should immediately report symptoms of toxicity, including diarrhea, vomiting, tremor, drowsiness, and muscle weakness.
- Adjust dose in renal impairment.
- Lithium levels may be increased by decreased salt intake, NSAIDs, ACEIs, ARBs, and metronidazole, and may be decreased by increased salt intake, caffeine, and theophylline.
- Take with food to decrease GI upset. Adequate sodium and fluid intake (2500-3500 mL) should be maintained, especially during stabilization period.
- Side effects: nausea, mild thirst, dehydration, hypotension

LORAZEPAM

Brand Name
- Ativan

Pharmacologic Class
- Benzodiazepine

Mechanism of Action
- Causes CNS depression by potentiating the effects of GABA (an inhibitory neurotransmitter).

Dosage Forms
- Oral (tablet, solution), injection solution (IM/IV)

Common Uses
- Treatment of anxiety disorders and status epilepticus (injection)

Quick Facts
- DEA Schedule IV
- Black Box Warning – Concomitant use with opioids increases risk of sedation, respiratory depression, coma, or death.
- Avoid abrupt discontinuation to prevent withdrawal symptoms.
- Avoid alcohol and other CNS depressants.
- Metabolized to inactive compounds, therefore it may be less harmful for elderly patients or patients with hepatic impairment.
- Side effects: drowsiness, dizziness, lightheadedness, ataxia

LOSARTAN

Brand Name
- Cozaar

Pharmacologic Class
- ARB

Mechanism of Action
- Blocks the binding of angiotensin II to the angiotensin II type-1 receptor on vascular smooth muscle, which prevents vasoconstriction and the secretion of aldosterone.

Dosage Form
- Oral (tablet)

Common Uses
- Treatment of hypertension and diabetic nephropathy; used to reduce the risk of stroke in patients with hypertension and left ventricular hypertrophy

Quick Facts
- Black Box Warning – Discontinue use as soon as possible if pregnancy is detected.
- Contraindicated with concomitant use with aliskiren in diabetic patients.
- NSAIDs may reduce antihypertensive effect and increase the risk of renal dysfunction.
- Patients should avoid potassium supplements or salt substitutes containing potassium without first consulting healthcare provider.
- Side effects: dizziness, cough, nasal congestion, upper respiratory tract infection

LOSARTAN-HYDROCHLOROTHIAZIDE

Brand Name
- Hyzaar

Pharmacologic Class
- Combination ARB and thiazide diuretic

Mechanism of Action
- Losartan blocks the binding of angiotensin II to the angiotensin II type-1 receptor on vascular smooth muscle, which prevents vasoconstriction and the secretion of aldosterone. Hydrochlorothiazide inhibits sodium and chloride reabsorption in the renal distal convoluted tubule.

Dosage Form
- Oral (tablet)

Common Uses
- Treatment of hypertension; used to reduce the risk of stroke in patients with hypertension and left ventricular hypertrophy

Quick Facts
- Black Box Warning – Discontinue use as soon as possible if pregnancy is detected.
- Contraindicated in patients with anuria, concomitant use with aliskiren in diabetic patients, and hypersensitivity to sulfonamides.
- Administer in the morning because of increased diuresis.
- Patients should avoid potassium supplements or salt substitutes containing potassium without first consulting healthcare provider.
- Side effects: dizziness, cough, upper respiratory tract infection, back pain

LOTEPREDNOL

Brand Names
- Lotemax, Alrex, Inveltys

Pharmacologic Class
- Corticosteroid

Mechanism of Action
- The anti-inflammatory effect is believed to be due to stimulation of phospholipase A_2 inhibitory proteins. These proteins subsequently block the release of arachidonic acid, which is a precursor to leukotrienes and prostaglandins.

Dosage Forms
- Ophthalmic (suspension, ointment, gel)

Common Uses
- Treatment of ophthalmic inflammation, post-operative ophthalmic inflammation and pain, and seasonal allergic conjunctivitis

Quick Facts
- Monitor intraocular pressure if medication is used for 10 days or longer. Prolonged use of corticosteroids may result in glaucoma with damage to the optic nerve, and defects in visual acuity and fields of vision.
- Patients using Lotemax should not wear contact lenses during therapy.
- Patients should remove contact lenses before instilling Inveltys and Alrex. Lenses may be reinserted 15 minutes after using Inveltys and 10 minutes after using Alrex.
- Side effects: ocular pain or discomfort, blurred vision, foreign body sensation

LOVASTATIN

Brand Names
- Mevacor, Altoprev

Pharmacologic Class
- HMG-CoA reductase inhibitor

Mechanism of Action
- Inhibits HMG-CoA reductase, preventing the conversion of HMG-CoA to mevalonate (the rate-limiting step in cholesterol synthesis).

Dosage Form
- Oral (tablet)

Common Use
- Treatment of hyperlipidemia

Quick Facts
- CYP3A4 inhibitors can increase plasma concentration of medication.
- Contraindicated in active liver disease and in pregnancy and lactation.
- Monitor LFTs at baseline and periodically thereafter.
- Limit alcohol intake and avoid grapefruit and grapefruit juice.
- Immediate-release tablet should be taken with evening meal. Extended-release tablet should be taken at bedtime.
- Side effects: diarrhea, constipation, increased liver enzymes, dyspepsia, arthralgia

LUBIPROSTONE

Brand Name
- Amitiza

Pharmacologic Class
- Chloride channel activator

Mechanism of Action
- Acts locally on the apical membrane of the gastrointestinal tract to increase intestinal fluid secretion and motility.

Dosage Form
- Oral (capsule)

Common Uses
- Treatment of chronic idiopathic constipation, irritable bowel syndrome with constipation in women ≥ 18 years old, and opioid-induced constipation in patients with chronic noncancer pain

Quick Facts
- Contraindicated in patients with known or suspected mechanical GI obstruction.
- Administer with food and water to decrease nausea.
- Patients may experience dyspnea within an hour of the first dose. The symptom usually resolves within 3 hours, but may recur with repeat dosing.
- Side effects: nausea, diarrhea, flatulence, abdominal pain, distension

LURASIDONE

Brand Name
- Latuda

Pharmacologic Class
- Antipsychotic

Mechanism of Action
- Blocks dopamine D_2 and serotonin 5-HT_{2A} receptors in the brain.

Dosage Form
- Oral (tablet)

Common Uses
- Treatment of schizophrenia and bipolar depression

Quick Facts
- Black Box Warnings – Elderly patients with dementia-related psychosis treated with antipsychotic drugs are at an increased risk of death. There is an increased risk of suicidal thoughts and behavior in pediatric and young adult patients.
- Concomitant use with a strong CYP3A4 inhibitor or CYP3A4 inducer is contraindicated.
- Avoid grapefruit and grapefruit juice.
- Can prolong the QT interval.
- Patients should be counseled to report signs of extrapyramidal symptoms (restlessness, tremor, stiffness, etc.) or neuroleptic malignant syndrome (sweating, fever, muscle rigidity, etc.).
- Medication should be administered with food to increase absorption (at least 350 calories).
- Monitor for hyperglycemia, dyslipidemia, and weight gain.
- Side effects: somnolence, nausea, extrapyramidal disorder, akathisia

MECLIZINE

Brand Name
▪ Antivert

Pharmacologic Class
▪ H_1 antagonist

Mechanism of Action
▪ Antagonist at H_1 receptors in the CNS that also has anticholinergic effects.

Dosage Forms
▪ Oral (tablet, chewable tablet)

Common Uses
▪ Treatment of vertigo; prevention and treatment of motion sickness

Quick Facts
▪ Use with caution in patients with asthma, BPH, and glaucoma.
▪ Avoid alcohol and other CNS depressants while taking medication.
▪ For the prevention of motion sickness, take 1 hour before departure. The dose may be repeated every 24 hours as necessary.
▪ Side effects: drowsiness, dry mouth, blurred vision, headache

MEDROXYPROGESTERONE ACETATE

Brand Names
- Depo-Provera, Provera

Pharmacologic Class
- Contraceptive and progestin

Mechanism of Action
- Medroxyprogesterone converts a proliferative endometrium into a secretory one. When administered parenterally, medroxyprogesterone inhibits the secretion of pituitary gonadotropins, which prevents follicular maturation and ovulation.

Dosage Forms
- Oral (tablet), injection suspension (IM/SubQ)

Common Uses
- Prevention of pregnancy; treatment of endometriosis-associated pain, abnormal uterine bleeding, and endometrial carcinoma; prevention of endometrial hyperplasia

Quick Facts
- Black Box Warnings (oral use) – Estrogen plus progestins should not be used for the prevention of cardiovascular disease. Increased risks of MI, stroke, invasive breast cancer, pulmonary emboli, and DVT in postmenopausal women (50 to 79 years of age) using estrogens combined with medroxyprogesterone acetate have been reported. An increased risk of developing probable dementia in postmenopausal women ≥ 65 years old has been reported when using estrogen plus progestin.
- Black Box Warnings (injectable) – Women who use medroxyprogesterone acetate injection may lose significant bone mineral density. Injection should not be used as a long-term birth control method (i.e., longer than 2 years) unless other methods are inadequate.
- Side effects: abnormal menstrual bleeding, weight gain, abdominal pain, headache

MELOXICAM

Brand Names
- Mobic, Vivlodex

Pharmacologic Class
- NSAID

Mechanism of Action
- Prevents the synthesis of prostaglandins by inhibiting the cyclooxygenase-1 and cyclooxygenase-2 (COX-1 and 2) enzymes.

Dosage Forms
- Oral (tablet, disintegrating tablet, capsule, suspension)

Common Uses
- Treatment of osteoarthritis and rheumatoid arthritis (disintegrating tablet and suspension only)

Quick Facts
- Black Box Warnings – Increased risk of cardiovascular thrombotic events and GI bleeding, ulceration, and perforation. Contraindicated in the setting of coronary artery bypass graft surgery.
- Contraindicated in patients with a history of asthma, urticaria, or other allergic-type reactions after taking aspirin or other NSAIDs.
- Pregnant patients should avoid use starting at 30 weeks gestation due to the risk of premature closure of the ductus arteriosus.
- Use with caution in patients with renal or hepatic impairment.
- Side effects: dyspepsia, nausea, diarrhea, constipation, abdominal pain

MEMANTINE

Brand Name
- Namenda

Pharmacologic Class
- NMDA receptor antagonist

Mechanism of Action
- Inhibits glutamate from binding to NMDA receptors, which decreases activation of NMDA receptors in the CNS.

Dosage Forms
- Oral (tablet, capsule, solution)

Common Use
- Treatment of Alzheimer's disease

Quick Facts
- Dosage in severe renal impairment (CrCl < 30 mL/min) should not exceed 5 mg twice daily (immediate release) or 14 mg once daily (extended release).
- Medications or genitourinary conditions that alkalinize the urine (carbonic anhydrase inhibitors, sodium bicarbonate, severe infection of the urinary tract, etc.) may increase plasma levels of memantine.
- Daily doses greater than 5 mg should be given twice per day and dose increases should not be titrated sooner than once per week.
- Side effects: confusion, dizziness, headache, fatigue

MESALAMINE

Brand Names
- Apriso, Lialda, Pentasa

Pharmacologic Class
- Aminosalicylate

Mechanism of Action
- Mechanism of action remains unknown, but may block cyclooxygenase and inhibit prostaglandin formation in the colon.

Dosage Forms
- Oral (tablet, capsule), rectal (suppository, enema)

Common Uses
- Treatment of mild to moderate ulcerative colitis, mild to moderate distal ulcerative colitis, proctosigmoiditis, and proctitis

Quick Facts
- Contraindicated in patients with a hypersensitivity to salicylates, including aspirin.
- Patients taking Apriso should avoid concomitant use with antacids.
- Suppositories can stain surfaces such as fabrics, granite, marble, etc.
- Medication may cause photosensitivity. Patients should limit sunlight and UV light exposure.
- Side effects when used rectally: dizziness, rectal pain, fever, rash, colitis
- Side effects when used orally: abdominal pain, nausea, vomiting, dizziness, headache

METAXALONE

Brand Name
- Skelaxin

Pharmacologic Class
- Skeletal muscle relaxant

Mechanism of Action
- Mechanism of action remains unknown, but may be due to general CNS depression. It has no direct action on the contractile mechanism of striated muscle, the motor end plate, or the nerve fiber.

Dosage Form
- Oral (tablet)

Common Use
- Treatment of acute musculoskeletal pain

Quick Facts
- Use is contraindicated in patients with significant renal or hepatic impairment. LFTs should be monitored periodically. Also contraindicated in patients with any type of anemia.
- Use with caution when taken concurrently with other CNS depressants.
- Medication can cause serotonin syndrome when taken at higher than recommended doses or when used concurrently with other serotonergic medications, including SSRIs, SNRIs, TCAs, triptans, etc.
- Avoid alcohol use.
- Side effects: GI discomfort, nausea, vomiting, nervousness, drowsiness

METFORMIN

Brand Names
- Glucophage, Glumetza

Pharmacologic Class
- Biguanide

Mechanism of Action
- Decreases hepatic glucose production and intestinal absorption of glucose, and improves insulin sensitivity by increasing peripheral glucose uptake and utilization.

Dosage Forms
- Oral (tablet, solution, suspension)

Common Use
- Treatment of type 2 diabetes

Quick Facts
- Black Box Warning – Metformin-associated lactic acidosis has resulted in death, hypothermia, hypotension, and resistant bradyarrhythmias. Risk factors include renal or hepatic impairment, age $\geq$ 65, having a radiologic study with contrast, surgery and other procedures, hypoxic states, and excessive alcohol intake.
- Contraindicated in severe renal impairment (eGFR < 30 mL/min/1.73m^2) and acute or chronic metabolic acidosis, including diabetic ketoacidosis.
- Medication can decrease folate and vitamin B_{12} absorption. Patients may need supplementation.
- Administer with food.
- Side effects: diarrhea, nausea, vomiting, unpleasant metallic taste

METFORMIN-GLYBURIDE

Brand Name
- Glucovance

Pharmacologic Class
- Combination biguanide and sulfonylurea

Mechanism of Action
- Metformin decreases hepatic glucose production and intestinal absorption of glucose and improves insulin sensitivity by increasing peripheral glucose uptake and utilization. Glyburide stimulates insulin release from pancreatic beta cells.

Dosage Form
- Oral (tablet)

Common Use
- Treatment of type 2 diabetes

Quick Facts
- Black Box Warning – Metformin-associated lactic acidosis has resulted in death, hypothermia, hypotension, and resistant bradyarrhythmias. (See "metformin" for additional details.)
- Contraindicated in severe renal impairment (eGFR < 30 mL/min/1.73m^2) and acute or chronic metabolic acidosis, including diabetic ketoacidosis.
- Can decrease folate and vitamin B$_{12}$ absorption. Patients may need supplementation.
- Administer with food.
- Patients should be counseled to monitor for signs of hypoglycemia (sweating, tremor, blurred vision, headache, etc.), and to always have a source of oral glucose available for treatment.
- Side effects: upper respiratory tract infection, diarrhea, abdominal pain, nausea, vomiting

METHADONE

Brand Names
- Dolophine, Methadose

Pharmacologic Class
- Opioid analgesic

Mechanism of Action
- Binds to the mu opioid receptor, which reduces neuronal cell excitability and transmission of nociceptive impulses. Methadone is also an NMDA receptor antagonist.

Dosage Forms
- Oral (tablet, solution), injection solution (IM/IV)

Common Uses
- Treatment of moderate to severe pain and opioid addiction

Quick Facts
- DEA Schedule II
- Black Box Warnings – QT interval prolongation and serious arrhythmias, including torsades de pointes, have occurred. Serious, life-threatening, or fatal respiratory depression may occur. Concomitant use with benzodiazepines increases risk of sedation, respiratory depression, coma, or death. Concomitant use with CYP3A4 inhibitors, or discontinuation of CYP3A4 inducers, can result in a fatal overdose of methadone. Prolonged use of methadone during pregnancy can result in neonatal opioid withdrawal syndrome.
- Side effects: sedation, constipation, pruritis, sweating, dry mouth

METHIMAZOLE

Brand Name
- Tapazole

Pharmacologic Class
- Antithyroid agent

Mechanism of Action
- Inhibits the synthesis of thyroxine (T_4) and triiodothyronine (T_3) by blocking the oxidation of iodine in the thyroid gland.

Dosage Form
- Oral (tablet)

Common Use
- Treatment of hyperthyroidism

Quick Facts
- Total daily dosage is usually given in 3 divided doses at 8-hour intervals.
- Medication can cause agranulocytosis and hepatotoxicity. CBC and LFTs should be performed prior to initiation of therapy.
- Can be taken with or without food but must be consistent.
- Side effects: rash, pruritis, nausea, vomiting

METHOCARBAMOL

Brand Name
- Robaxin

Pharmacologic Class
- Skeletal muscle relaxant

Mechanism of Action
- Mechanism of action remains unknown, but may be due to general CNS depression. It has no direct action on the contractile mechanism of striated muscle, the motor end plate, or the nerve fiber.

Dosage Forms
- Oral (tablet), injection solution (IM/IV)

Common Use
- Treatment of skeletal muscle spasm associated with acute, painful musculoskeletal conditions

Quick Facts
- Medication may be administered with or without food, but serum concentrations may be increased when taken with food.
- Injection form can cause extravasation. Patients should be placed in a recumbent position during and for 10 to 15 minutes after IV administration.
- Use with caution when taken concurrently with other CNS depressants.
- Abrupt discontinuation of long-term therapy may cause withdrawal symptoms.
- Avoid alcohol use.
- Side effects: dizziness, drowsiness, rash, pruritis, nausea

METHOTREXATE

Brand Names
- Trexall, Rheumatrex

Pharmacologic Class
- Antimetabolite

Mechanism of Action
- Methotrexate inhibits dihydrofolate reductase (DHFR), which interferes with DNA synthesis, repair, and cellular replication. The mechanism of action in rheumatoid arthritis is unknown. In psoriasis, methotrexate targets rapidly proliferating epithelial cells in the skin.

Dosage Forms
- Oral (tablet, solution), injection (solution)

Common Uses
- Treatment of certain types of cancer, rheumatoid arthritis, psoriasis, and psoriatic arthritis

Quick Facts
- Black Box Warnings – Death, fetal death and/or congenital abnormalities, lung disease, tumor lysis syndrome, fatal skin reactions, and *Pneumocystis jiroveci* pneumonia have been reported. Monitor for bone marrow, liver, lung, and kidney toxicities. Hepatotoxicity, fibrosis, and cirrhosis occur with prolonged use. Diarrhea and ulcerative stomatitis require interruption of therapy.
- Patient should maintain adequate hydration during therapy to minimize renal toxicity.
- Medications that interfere with methotrexate clearance include NSAIDs, penicillins, and probenecid. Avoid concurrent use.
- High doses of methotrexate require leucovorin to decrease toxicity.
- Side effects: diarrhea, nausea, vomiting, rash, thrombocytopenia, hand-foot syndrome

METHYLPHENIDATE

Brand Names
- Ritalin, Concerta, Metadate ER

Pharmacologic Class
- CNS stimulant

Mechanism of Action
- Believed to block the reuptake of norepinephrine and dopamine in presynaptic nerve endings.

Dosage Forms
- Oral (tablet, chewable tablet, capsule, solution, powder for suspension), transdermal (patch)

Common Uses
- Treatment of ADHD and narcolepsy

Quick Facts
- DEA Schedule II
- Black Box Warning – High potential for abuse, and administration for prolonged periods of time may lead to dependence. Misuse may cause sudden death and serious cardiovascular adverse reactions.
- Use is contraindicated during or within 14 days of MAOI administration.
- Gradually increase dosing and avoid abrupt discontinuation to prevent withdrawal symptoms.
- Maximum wear time for patch is 9 hours/day. Do not expose patch to external heat sources.
- Side effects: decreased appetite, weight loss, nausea, insomnia, headache

METHYLPREDNISOLONE

Brand Name
- Medrol

Pharmacologic Class
- Corticosteroid

Mechanism of Action
- Binds to cytoplasmic receptors in cells. The steroid-receptor complex then enters the nucleus of cells where it modifies transcription and thus the synthesis of proteins and enzymes involved with inflammation.

Dosage Form
- Oral (tablet)

Common Uses
- Treatment of various allergic and inflammatory diseases, including endocrine disorders, respiratory diseases, rheumatic disorders, etc.

Quick Facts
- Patients on long-term therapy should avoid live or live-attenuated vaccines due to drug-induced immunosuppression.
- Take with food to decrease GI upset.
- Contraindicated in patients with systemic fungal infections because the infections may be exacerbated.
- Has low sodium-retaining potential.
- Taper dose to prevent withdrawal symptoms if used longer than 2 weeks.
- Short-term side effects: insomnia, stomach upset, fluid retention, increased appetite
- Long-term side effects: Cushing's syndrome, osteoporosis, muscle wasting, growth suppression in children

METOCLOPRAMIDE

Brand Name
- Reglan

Pharmacologic Class
- Dopamine antagonist

Mechanism of Action
- Antiemetic effect is due to inhibition of dopamine D_2 and serotonin 5-HT_3 receptors in the chemoreceptor trigger zone of the CNS. Antagonism of D_2 receptors also enhances cholinergic stimulation of smooth muscle, which increases lower esophageal sphincter tone and accelerates gastric emptying and intestinal transit.

Dosage Forms
- Oral (tablet, disintegrating tablet, solution), injection solution (IM/IV)

Common Uses
- Treatment of diabetic gastroparesis and refractory GERD; prophylaxis of chemotherapy-induced nausea and vomiting and postoperative nausea and vomiting

Quick Facts
- Black Box Warning – Tardive dyskinesia (TD) can occur, which is often irreversible. Metoclopramide should be discontinued in patients who develop signs or symptoms of TD. Duration of treatment with metoclopramide should not exceed 12 weeks.
- Oral dosage forms should be administered 30 minutes before meals and at bedtime or as a single dose prior to a provoking situation.
- Avoid concomitant use with MAOIs, tricyclic antidepressants, or sympathomimetic amines.
- Risk of QT interval prolongation.
- Side effects: restlessness, drowsiness, fluid retention, fatigue

METOPROLOL

Brand Names
- Lopressor (metoprolol tartrate), Toprol XL (metoprolol succinate)

Pharmacologic Class
- Beta$_1$-selective blocker

Mechanism of Action
- Binds to the beta$_1$-adrenergic receptors found in vascular smooth muscle and the heart, blocking the positive inotropic and chronotropic actions of endogenous catecholamines such as isoproterenol, norepinephrine, and epinephrine.

Dosage Forms
- Tartrate: Oral (tablet, powder for solution), intravenous (solution)
- Succinate: Oral (tablet, capsule)

Common Uses
- Treatment of hypertension, angina pectoris (chronic), acute MI (tartrate), and congestive heart failure (succinate)

Quick Facts
- Black Box Warning – Abrupt cessation may precipitate angina, MI, arrhythmias, or rebound hypertension.
- Contraindications include AV block, bradycardia, cardiogenic shock, and overt heart failure.
- Medication can mask symptoms of hypoglycemia in diabetics.
- Take with food to increase absorption.
- Side effects: bradycardia, hypotension, dizziness, fatigue

METRONIDAZOLE

Brand Names
- Flagyl, Metrocream, Metrogel

Pharmacologic Class
- Antibiotic

Mechanism of Action
- Inhibits protein synthesis by interacting with DNA and causing a loss of helical DNA structure and strand breakage.

Dosage Forms
- Oral (tablet, capsule), topical (cream, lotion, vaginal gel), intravenous (solution)

Common Uses
- Treatment of intestinal amebiasis, bacterial meningitis, intra-abdominal infections, bacterial vaginosis, and rosacea

Quick Facts
- Black Box Warning – May be carcinogenic based on some animal studies in mice and rats. The use of metronidazole should be reserved only for conditions approved by the FDA.
- Patients should avoid consuming alcohol or products containing propylene glycol while taking metronidazole and for at least 3 days afterward. Abdominal cramps, nausea, vomiting, headaches, and flushing may occur.
- Metronidazole should not be used concomitantly or within 2 weeks of disulfiram.
- Immediate-release tablets may be taken with food or milk if GI upset occurs. Extended-release tablets should be taken at least 1 hour before or 2 hours after a meal.
- Side effects: diarrhea, nausea, vomiting, metallic taste, peripheral neuropathy

MINOCYCLINE (systemic)

Brand Names
- Minocin, Solodyn

Pharmacologic Class
- Tetracycline antibiotic

Mechanism of Action
- Inhibits bacterial protein synthesis by binding to the 30S ribosomal subunit.

Dosage Forms
- Oral (tablet, capsule), intravenous (powder for solution)

Common Uses
- Treatment of acne, Rocky Mountain spotted fever, and respiratory tract infections caused by *Myocoplasma pneumoniae*

Quick Facts
- Medication should be administered with at least 8 oz. of water to prevent esophageal irritation or ulceration.
- Medication can cause photosensitivity. Patients should use sunscreen and avoid prolonged exposure to sunlight and tanning beds.
- Can cause permanent discoloration of teeth and should not be used during tooth development (last half of pregnancy, infancy, and children ≤ 8 years old).
- Avoid concomitant oral use with iron or antacids containing aluminum, calcium, or magnesium.
- Side effects: diarrhea, nausea, dizziness, photosensitivity

MIRTAZAPINE

Brand Name
- Remeron

Pharmacologic Class
- Tetracyclic antidepressant

Mechanism of Action
- Increases the release of norepinephrine and serotonin through antagonist activity of central presynaptic alpha$_2$-adrenergic receptors. Mirtazapine is also an antagonist at serotonin 5-HT$_2$ and 5-HT$_3$ receptors, alpha$_1$-adrenergic receptors, histamine H$_1$ receptors, and muscarinic receptors.

Dosage Forms
- Oral (tablet, disintegrating tablet)

Common Use
- Treatment of depression

Quick Facts
- Black Box Warning – Increased risk of suicidal thoughts and behavior in children, adolescents, and young adults.
- Use is contraindicated during or within 14 days of MAOI administration.
- May cause QT prolongation.
- Should be administered at bedtime due to sedation.
- Side effects: drowsiness, increased appetite, weight gain, dry mouth, constipation

MODAFINIL

Brand Name
- Provigil

Pharmacologic Class
- CNS stimulant

Mechanism of Action
- Mechanism of action remains unknown. Modafinil has been shown to inhibit the reuptake of dopamine by blocking dopamine transporters, and also decrease GABA-mediated neurotransmission.

Dosage Form
- Oral (tablet)

Common Uses
- Improves wakefulness in adult patients with narcolepsy, obstructive sleep apnea, and shift work sleep disorder

Quick Facts
- DEA Schedule IV
- Medication should be discontinued at the first sign of rash, unless the rash is clearly not drug related. Serious rash, including Stevens-Johnson syndrome, toxic epidermal necrolysis, and drug rash with eosinophilia and systemic symptoms have occurred during treatment.
- For patients with narcolepsy or obstructive sleep apnea, take in the morning. For patients with shift work disorder, take 1 hour before work shift.
- May decrease plasma levels of ethinyl estradiol during concomitant use and for 1 month after discontinuation. Alternative or concomitant contraception methods are recommended.
- Side effects: anxiety, insomnia, nausea, headache

MOMETASONE

Brand Names
- Nasonex, Asmanex, Elocon

Pharmacologic Class
- Corticosteroid

Mechanism of Action
- Inhibits inflammatory cells (mast cells, eosinophils, basophils, lymphocytes, macrophages, and neutrophils) and release of inflammatory mediators (histamine, eicosanoids, leukotrienes, and cytokines).

Dosage Forms
- Nasal (suspension), inhalation (powder, aerosol powder), topical (cream)

Common Uses
- Treatment of allergic rhinitis and nasal polyps (nasal dosage form), asthma (inhalation dosage forms), and corticosteroid-responsive dermatoses (topical dosage form)

Quick Facts
- Nasal spray may take several days of regular use for rhinitis symptoms to improve, and maximum benefit may take 1 to 2 weeks.
- Patients using inhalation dosage forms should rinse mouth with water, without swallowing, after each use to prevent oral candidiasis.
- Avoid using topical dosage forms with occlusive dressings unless directed by prescriber. Do not use on face, axillae, or groin.
- Side effects with nasal use: epistaxis, cough, headache
- Side effects with inhalation use: nasopharyngitis, headache, sinusitis, influenza
- Side effects with topical use: skin atrophy, burning, pruritis

MOMETASONE-FORMOTEROL

Brand Name
- Dulera

Pharmacologic Class
- Combination corticosteroid and beta$_2$-agonist

Mechanism of Action
- Mometasone inhibits inflammatory cells (mast cells, eosinophils, basophils, lymphocytes, macrophages, and neutrophils) and release of inflammatory mediators (histamine, eicosanoids, leukotrienes, and cytokines). Formoterol binds to beta$_2$-receptors and increases the level of cAMP, which relaxes bronchial smooth muscle.

Dosage Form
- Inhalation (aerosol powder)

Common Use
- Treatment of asthma

Quick Facts
- Prime inhaler prior to first use and if it has not been used for more than 5 days.
- If using 2 inhalations per dose, wait at least 30 seconds before taking second puff.
- Clean mouthpiece with a dry wipe every 7 days.
- Counsel patients to rinse mouth with water, without swallowing, after each use to prevent oral candidiasis.
- Side effects: upper respiratory tract infection, nasopharyngitis, sinusitis, headache

MONTELUKAST

Brand Name
- Singulair

Pharmacologic Class
- Leukotriene receptor antagonist

Mechanism of Action
- Binds to the cysteinyl leukotriene receptor type-1 receptors in the airway (including airway smooth muscle cells and airway macrophages), which prevents airway edema, smooth muscle contraction, and airway inflammation.

Dosage Forms
- Oral (tablet, chewable tablet, granules)

Common Uses
- Prophylaxis and chronic treatment of asthma; prophylaxis of exercise-induced asthma; treatment of seasonal and perennial allergic rhinitis

Quick Facts
- Black Box Warning – Serious neuropsychiatric events that may include suicidal thoughts or actions, or completed suicides, have been reported during treatment and after discontinuation in patients with and without pre-existing psychiatric disease.
- Montelukast is not for the treatment of acute asthma attacks.
- Avoid concomitant use with aspirin or NSAIDs in aspirin-sensitive patients.
- Chewable tablets contain phenylalanine.
- Side effects: upper respiratory tract infection, fever, headache, cough, abdominal pain

MORPHINE

Brand Names
- MS Contin, Kadian, Roxanol

Pharmacologic Class
- Opioid analgesic

Mechanism of Action
- Binds to the mu opioid receptor, which reduces neuronal cell excitability and transmission of nociceptive impulses.

Dosage Forms
- Oral (tablet, capsule, solution), injection solution (IM/IV), rectal (suppository)

Common Use
- Treatment of moderate to severe pain

Quick Facts
- DEA Schedule II
- Black Box Warnings – Serious, life-threatening, or fatal respiratory depression may occur. Concomitant use with benzodiazepines increases risk of sedation, respiratory depression, coma, or death. Prolonged use of morphine during pregnancy can result in neonatal opioid withdrawal syndrome.
- Contraindications include acute or severe bronchial asthma.
- Do not break, chew, or crush long-acting forms.
- Avoid abrupt discontinuation to prevent withdrawal symptoms.
- Side effects: somnolence, constipation, pruritus, dry mouth, sweating

MOXIFLOXACIN (systemic)

Brand Name
- Avelox

Pharmacologic Class
- Fluoroquinolone antibiotic

Mechanism of Action
- Prevents the synthesis of bacterial DNA by inhibiting DNA gyrase (topoisomerase II) and topoisomerase IV.

Dosage Forms
- Oral (tablet), intravenous (solution)

Common Uses
- Treatment of community-acquired pneumonia, skin and skin structure infections, exacerbation of acute bronchitis, sinusitis

Quick Facts
- Black Box Warnings – Risk of tendinitis, tendon rupture, peripheral neuropathy, CNS effects, and exacerbation of myasthenia gravis.
- Take medication 4 hours before or 8 hours after aluminum or magnesium-containing antacids or products containing calcium, iron, or zinc.
- May cause QT prolongation.
- Diabetic patients should carefully monitor blood glucose.
- Drink plenty of fluids to prevent crystalluria.
- Side effects: nausea, rash, diarrhea, sun sensitivity

MUPIROCIN

Brand Names
- Bactroban, Centany

Pharmacologic Class
- Topical antibiotic

Mechanism of Action
- Inhibits bacterial protein synthesis by binding to isoleucyl transfer-RNA synthetase.

Dosage Forms
- Topical (ointment, cream)

Common Uses
- Treatment of impetigo due to *S. aureus* and *S. Pyogenes* (ointment), treatment of secondary infected traumatic skin lesions due to *S. aureus* and *S. Pyogenes* (cream), prophylaxis and treatment of MRSA infections in the nasal cavity (ointment)

Quick Facts
- For intranasal ointment, apply inside nostrils, press sides of nose together, and gently massage the nostrils for about 1 minute to spread the ointment throughout the nostrils. Do not use with any other nasal preparations.
- Apply a small amount of ointment or cream to the affected area. The area may be covered with a gauze dressing unless patient was instructed by prescriber to leave it uncovered. Do not use with any other lotions, creams, or ointments.
- Patient should contact prescriber if no improvement is seen in 3 to 5 days.
- Side effects: application site pain, burning, or stinging. Nasal ointment may also cause headache and taste disturbances.

MYCOPHENOLATE MOFETIL

Brand Name
- CellCept

Pharmacologic Class
- Immunosuppressant

Mechanism of Action
- Mycophenolate mofetil is a prodrug of mycophenolic acid (MPA), which inhibits inosine monophosphate dehydrogenase. MPA depletes guanosine nucleotides in T and B lymphocytes and inhibits their proliferation.

Dosage Forms
- Oral (tablet, capsule, powder for suspension), intravenous (powder for solution)

Common Uses
- Prophylaxis of organ rejection in renal, cardiac, and hepatic transplants

Quick Facts
- Black Box Warnings – Increased risk of developing lymphomas and other malignancies, particularly of the skin; increased susceptibility to infection, including opportunistic infections, fatal infections, and sepsis. Use during pregnancy is associated with increased risks of first trimester pregnancy loss and congenital malformations.
- CellCept should be used concomitantly with cyclosporine and corticosteroids.
- Take oral dosage forms on an empty stomach, either 1 hour before or 2 hours after a meal. In stable kidney transplant patients, CellCept can be taken with food if necessary.
- Do not administer simultaneously with antacids.
- Side effects: diarrhea, abdominal pain, vomiting, edema, hypertension

NABUMETONE

Brand Name
- Relafen

Pharmacologic Class
- NSAID

Mechanism of Action
- Prevents the synthesis of prostaglandins by inhibiting the cyclooxygenase-1 and cyclooxygenase-2 (COX-1 and 2) enzymes.

Dosage Form
- Oral (tablet)

Common Uses
- Treatment of osteoarthritis and rheumatoid arthritis

Quick Facts
- Black Box Warnings – Increased risk of cardiovascular thrombotic events and GI bleeding, ulceration, and perforation. Contraindicated in the setting of coronary artery bypass graft surgery.
- Contraindicated in patients with a history of asthma, urticaria, or other allergic-type reactions after taking aspirin or other NSAIDs.
- Pregnant patients should avoid use starting in the third trimester due to the risk of premature closure of the ductus arteriosus.
- Use with caution in patients with renal or hepatic impairment.
- Side effects: dyspepsia, diarrhea, abdominal pain, tinnitus, edema, pruritis

NAPROXEN

Brand Name
- Naprosyn

Pharmacologic Class
- NSAID

Mechanism of Action
- Prevents the synthesis of prostaglandins by inhibiting the cyclooxygenase-1 and cyclooxygenase-2 (COX-1 and 2) enzymes.

Dosage Forms
- Oral (tablet, capsule, suspension)

Common Uses
- Treatment of mild to moderate pain, osteoarthritis, rheumatoid arthritis, gout, dysmenorrhea, bursitis, tendinitis, and ankylosing spondylitis

Quick Facts
- Black Box Warnings – Increased risk of cardiovascular thrombotic events and GI bleeding, ulceration, and perforation. Contraindicated in the setting of coronary artery bypass graft surgery.
- Contraindicated in patients with a history of asthma, urticaria, or other allergic-type reactions after taking aspirin or other NSAIDs.
- Pregnant patients should avoid use starting at 30 weeks gestation due to the risk of premature closure of the ductus arteriosus.
- Use with caution in patients with renal or hepatic impairment.
- Side effects: heartburn, constipation, abdominal pain, edema, tinnitus, headache

NEBIVOLOL

Brand Name
- Bystolic

Pharmacologic Class
- $Beta_1$-selective blocker

Mechanism of Action
- Binds to the $beta_1$-adrenergic receptors found in vascular smooth muscle and the heart, blocking the positive inotropic and chronotropic actions of endogenous catecholamines such as isoproterenol, norepinephrine, and epinephrine. Also exerts nitric oxide-mediated vasodilation which decreases systemic vascular resistance.

Dosage Form
- Oral (tablet)

Common Use
- Treatment of hypertension

Quick Facts
- Contraindications include severe bradycardia, 2nd or 3rd degree AV block, cardiogenic shock, and severe hepatic impairment.
- Do not abruptly discontinue because it may exacerbate angina pectoris or cause MI or ventricular arrhythmias.
- Medication can mask symptoms of hypoglycemia in diabetics.
- Side effects: dizziness, headache, fatigue, nausea

NEOMYCIN-POLYMYXIN B-HYDROCORTISONE (otic)

Brand Names
- Cortisporin, Cortomycin

Pharmacologic Class
- Combination antibiotic and corticosteroid

Mechanism of Action
- Neomycin inhibits bacterial protein synthesis by binding to the 30S ribosomal subunit. Polymyxin B increases bacterial cell wall permeability, causing leakage of intracellular contents. Hydrocortisone has anti-inflammatory, antipruritic, and vasoconstrictive properties. The anti-inflammatory effect is believed to be due to stimulation of phospholipase A_2 inhibitory proteins. These proteins subsequently block the release of arachidonic acid, which is a precursor to leukotrienes and prostaglandins.

Dosage Forms
- Otic (solution, suspension)

Common Uses
- Treatment of acute otitis externa and infections of the mastoidectomy and fenestration cavities

Quick Facts
- Do not use for more than 10 consecutive days unless directed by prescriber.
- To instill drops, warm bottle in hands for 1 to 2 minutes (cold suspension can cause dizziness). Shake bottle gently. Lie down or tilt head so that affected ear faces upward. Straighten the ear canal by pulling earlobe up and back for adults or down and back for children. Instill the prescribed number of drops into the ear canal. Keep the ear facing up for 5 minutes.
- Side effects: ear itching, burning, irritation

NIACIN

Brand Names
▪ Niaspan, Niacor

Pharmacologic Class
▪ Antihyperlipidemic

Mechanism of Action
▪ Exact mechanism of action for antihyperlipidemic effect is unknown. It may involve several actions such as increased activity of lipoprotein lipase, decreased lipolysis in adipose tissue, and decreased esterification of hepatic triglycerides, which results in a decrease in VLDL, LDL, and triglycerides and an increase in HDL.

Dosage Forms
▪ Oral (tablet, capsule)

Common Uses
▪ Treatment of hyperlipidemia and hypertriglyceridemia; used to lower the risk of recurrent MI in patients with a history of MI and hyperlipidemia; used to slow progression or promote regression of coronary artery disease

Quick Facts
▪ Take at bedtime with a low-fat snack.
▪ Use with caution in patients predisposed to gout because it may increase uric acid.
▪ May increase fasting blood glucose, therefore monitoring is recommended.
▪ Monitor LFTs at baseline, every 6 to 12 weeks for the first year, then approximately every 6 months thereafter.
▪ Flushing is a common side effect that usually subsides after a few weeks of consistent therapy. Taking aspirin (up to 325 mg) or an NSAID 30 minutes before dose can minimize flushing.
▪ Side effects: flushing, pruritis, diarrhea, nausea, vomiting, GI distress

NIFEDIPINE

Brand Names
- Procardia, Adalat CC, Nifedical XL

Pharmacologic Class
- Calcium channel blocker

Mechanism of Action
- Dihydropyridine CCB that blocks the transmembrane influx of calcium ions into vascular smooth muscle and cardiac muscle which results in increased peripheral arterial vasodilation and decreased peripheral vascular resistance.

Dosage Forms
- Oral (tablet, capsule)

Common Uses
- Treatment of chronic stable angina, variant angina, and hypertension

Quick Facts
- May worsen angina and increase the risk of MI after starting or increasing dose.
- Take extended-release tablets on an empty stomach.
- Avoid grapefruit and grapefruit juice while taking medication.
- Do not abruptly discontinue medication.
- Side effects: peripheral edema, flushing, headache, palpitations

NITROFURANTOIN

Brand Names
- Macrobid, Macrodantin, Furadantin

Pharmacologic Class
- Antibiotic

Mechanism of Action
- Nitrofurantoin is reduced by bacterial flavoproteins to reactive intermediates which inactivate or alter bacterial ribosomal proteins and other macromolecules, resulting in inhibition of protein synthesis, aerobic energy metabolism, DNA, RNA, and cell wall synthesis.

Dosage Forms
- Oral (capsule, suspension)

Common Uses
- Prophylaxis and treatment of UTIs

Quick Facts
- Contraindications include anuria, significant renal impairment (CrCl < 60 mL/min), and pregnancy at term (38 to 42 weeks gestation).
- Administer with food to increase absorption.
- Avoid concomitant use with antacids containing magnesium trisilicate because it reduces the rate and extent of absorption of nitrofurantoin.
- Acute, subacute, and chronic pulmonary toxicity may occur. Patients should report symptoms of cough, malaise, dyspnea on exertion, and altered pulmonary function.
- Side effects: loss of appetite, nausea, vomiting, discoloration of the urine

NITROGLYCERIN

Brand Names
- Nitrostat, Nitro-Bid, Nitro-Dur

Pharmacologic Class
- Vasodilator

Mechanism of Action
- Acts as a prodrug for nitric oxide, which relaxes vascular smooth muscle and causes dilation of peripheral veins and arteries, with more prominent effects on veins to decrease cardiac preload.

Dosage Forms
- Oral (sublingual tablet, sublingual spray, sublingual powder, capsule), topical (ointment, rectal ointment), transdermal (patch), intravenous (solution)

Common Uses
- Prevention and treatment of angina pectoris; treatment of moderate to severe pain with chronic anal fissure (rectal ointment)

Quick Facts
- Patients using the sublingual tablets should be counseled to keep tablets in the original amber glass container, and that they expire by the expiration date printed on the bottle by the manufacturer. The tablets should be placed under the tongue or in the buccal pouch to dissolve—they should not be chewed or swallowed. Patients should contact EMS after taking 3 doses.
- Patients using the transdermal patch, ointment, or extended-release capsule dosage forms should allow a drug-free interval of 10 to 12 hours per day to prevent nitrate tolerance.
- Avoid concomitant use with PDE-5 inhibitors due to the risk of severe hypotension, syncope, or myocardial ischemia.
- Side effects: headache, dizziness, flushing, lightheadedness

NORETHINDRONE

Brand Names
- Ortho Micronor, Errin

Pharmacologic Class
- Oral contraceptive

Mechanism of Action
- Suppresses the production of luteinizing hormone and follicle-stimulating hormone, which prevents ovulation and alters cervical mucus and the endometrial lining.

Dosage Form
- Oral (tablet)

Common Use
- Prevention of pregnancy

Quick Facts
- Contraindications include breast cancer, active liver disease, and benign or malignant liver tumors.
- Medications that decrease the effectiveness of norethindrone include rifampin and St. John's wort.
- Take medication at the same time every day with no more than 24 hours between doses. If dose is more than 3 hours late or one or more pills are missed, take missed dose as soon as possible and use non-hormonal backup contraception for next 48 hours.
- Preferred for breastfeeding women. Women fully breastfeeding may start pills 6 weeks after delivery. Women partially breastfeeding may start pills 3 weeks after delivery.
- Side effects: headache, nausea, breast tenderness, menstrual irregularity

NORTRIPTYLINE

Brand Name
- Pamelor

Pharmacologic Class
- Tricyclic antidepressant

Mechanism of Action
- Increases the synaptic concentration of serotonin and norepinephrine in the CNS by inhibiting their reuptake at presynaptic nerve terminals. Also inhibits the action of histamine and acetylcholine.

Dosage Forms
- Oral (capsule, solution)

Common Use
- Treatment of depression

Quick Facts
- Black Box Warning – Increased risk of suicidal thoughts and behavior in children, adolescents, and young adults.
- Can prolong the QT interval.
- Use is contraindicated during or within 14 days of MAOI administration.
- Do not abruptly discontinue medication.
- Avoid alcohol use.
- Side effects: dry mouth, nausea, constipation, dizziness, weight gain

NYSTATIN

Brand Names
- Mycostatin, Nystop, Nyamyc

Pharmacologic Class
- Antifungal

Mechanism of Action
- Binds to sterols in the fungal cell membrane, which changes the permeability of the cell wall allowing leakage of cellular contents.

Dosage Forms
- Oral (tablet, suspension), topical (cream, ointment, powder)

Common Uses
- Treatment of oropharyngeal candidiasis (thrush), intestinal candidiasis, cutaneous and mucocutaneous candidiasis

Quick Facts
- Shake suspension well before using. Can be dosed as "swish and spit" for oral candidiasis or "swish and swallow" for esophageal candidiasis.
- Avoid using topical dosage forms with occlusive dressings unless directed by prescriber.
- Side effects from oral use: diarrhea, nausea, vomiting, facial swelling
- Side effects from topical use: burning, itching, rash

OFLOXACIN

Brand Names
- Ocuflox, Floxin

Pharmacologic Class
- Fluoroquinolone antibiotic

Mechanism of Action
- Prevents the synthesis of bacterial DNA by inhibiting DNA gyrase (topoisomerase II) and topoisomerase IV.

Dosage Forms
- Oral (tablet), ophthalmic (solution), otic (solution)

Common Uses
- Treatment of community-acquired pneumonia, acute exacerbation of chronic bronchitis, UTIs, skin and skin structure infections, bacterial conjunctivitis, corneal ulcers, acute otitis media, and otitis externa

Quick Facts
- Black Box Warnings (oral tablet) – Risk of tendinitis, tendon rupture, peripheral neuropathy, CNS effects, and exacerbation of myasthenia gravis.
- Take oral tablet 2 hours before or 2 hours after aluminum or magnesium-containing antacids or products containing calcium, iron, or zinc.
- Oral tablet may cause QT prolongation.
- Drink plenty of fluids when using oral tablets to prevent crystalluria.
- Diabetic patients should carefully monitor blood glucose.
- To instill otic drops, warm bottle in hands for 1 to 2 minutes (cold solution can cause dizziness).
- Side effects (oral): nausea, rash, diarrhea, sun sensitivity
- Side effects (otic): taste perversion, earache, pruritis
- Side effects (ophthalmic): burning, blurred vision, eye pain

OLANZAPINE

Brand Name
- Zyprexa

Pharmacologic Class
- Antipsychotic

Mechanism of Action
- Blocks dopamine D_2 and serotonin 5-HT_{2A} receptors in the brain.

Dosage Forms
- Oral (tablet, disintegrating tablet), intramuscular (powder for solution)

Common Uses
- Treatment of schizophrenia and bipolar disorder

Quick Facts
- Black Box Warning – Elderly patients with dementia-related psychosis treated with antipsychotics are at an increased risk of death compared to placebo. Most deaths appeared to be either cardiovascular (e.g., heart failure, sudden death) or infectious (e.g., pneumonia) in nature.
- Can prolong the QT interval.
- Patients should be counseled to report signs of extrapyramidal symptoms (restlessness, tremor, stiffness, etc.) or neuroleptic malignant syndrome (sweating, fever, muscle rigidity, etc.).
- Monitor for hyperglycemia, dyslipidemia, and weight gain.
- Side effects: somnolence, orthostatic hypotension, constipation, akathisia

OLMESARTAN

Brand Name
- Benicar

Pharmacologic Class
- ARB

Mechanism of Action
- Blocks the binding of angiotensin II to the angiotensin II type-1 receptor on vascular smooth muscle, which prevents vasoconstriction and the secretion of aldosterone.

Dosage Form
- Oral (tablet)

Common Use
- Treatment of hypertension

Quick Facts
- Black Box Warning – Discontinue use as soon as possible if pregnancy is detected.
- Contraindicated with concomitant use with aliskiren in diabetic patients.
- NSAIDs may reduce antihypertensive effect and increase the risk of renal dysfunction.
- Patients should avoid potassium supplements or salt substitutes containing potassium without first consulting healthcare provider.
- Side effects: dizziness, headache, diarrhea, rhinitis

OLMESARTAN-HYDROCHLOROTHIAZIDE

Brand Name
- Benicar HCT

Pharmacologic Class
- Combination ARB and thiazide diuretic

Mechanism of Action
- Olmesartan blocks the binding of angiotensin II to the angiotensin II type-1 receptor on vascular smooth muscle, which prevents vasoconstriction and the secretion of aldosterone. Hydrochlorothiazide inhibits sodium and chloride reabsorption in the renal distal convoluted tubule.

Dosage Form
- Oral (tablet)

Common Use
- Treatment of hypertension

Quick Facts
- Black Box Warning – Discontinue use as soon as possible if pregnancy is detected.
- Contraindicated in patients with anuria, concomitant use with aliskiren in diabetic patients, and hypersensitivity to sulfonamides.
- Administer in the morning because of increased diuresis.
- Patients should avoid potassium supplements or salt substitutes containing potassium without first consulting healthcare provider.
- Side effects: dizziness, nausea, hyperuricemia, upper respiratory tract infection

OLOPATADINE

Brand Names
- Patanol, Pataday, Pazeo, Patanase

Pharmacologic Class
- H_1 antagonist

Mechanism of Action
- H_1 antagonist that inhibits the release of histamine from mast cells

Dosage Forms
- Ophthalmic (solution), nasal (solution)

Common Uses
- Treatment of allergic conjunctivitis (ophthalmic) and allergic rhinitis (nasal)

Quick Facts
- Allow at least 10 minutes after using ophthalmic solution before inserting contact lenses.
- Nasal solution may cause epistaxis, nasal ulceration, and nasal septal perforation.
- Avoid alcohol and other CNS depressants when using nasal solution due to additive sedation.
- Side effects of ophthalmic solution: blurred vision, dry eye, dysgeusia, rhinitis, pharyngitis
- Side effects of nasal solution: bitter taste, post-nasal drip, cough, headache

OMEGA-3-ACID ETHYL ESTERS

Brand Name
- Lovaza

Pharmacologic Class
- Antihyperlipidemic

Mechanism of Action
- Reduces hepatic production of triglycerides, but mechanism of action is not completely understood. Possible mechanisms include inhibition of acyl-CoA:1,2-diacylglycerol acyltransferase, increased mitochondrial and peroxisomal β-oxidation in the liver, decreased lipogenesis in the liver, and increased plasma lipoprotein lipase activity.

Dosage Form
- Oral (capsule)

Common Use
- Treatment of hypertriglyceridemia

Quick Facts
- Use with caution in patients allergic to fish and/or shellfish.
- May be taken with or without food, but may be more comfortable to take with food.
- May increase bleeding times. Use with caution with anticoagulant and antiplatelets.
- May increase LDL. Monitor levels during therapy.
- Side effects: burping, dyspepsia, taste perversion, diarrhea

OMEPRAZOLE

Brand Name
- Prilosec

Pharmacologic Class
- PPI

Mechanism of Action
- Suppresses gastric acid secretion by inhibiting the H^+/K^+-ATPase pump in parietal cells, blocking the final step of acid production.

Dosage Forms
- Oral (tablet, capsule, powder for suspension)

Common Uses
- Treatment of GERD, erosive esophagitis, *H. pylori* eradication, peptic ulcer disease, and Zollinger-Ellison syndrome

Quick Facts
- Take at least 30 to 60 minutes before eating.
- Do not abruptly discontinue. Medication should be tapered to avoid acid rebound.
- Strong CYP2C19 inhibitor.
- Use with caution with other medications that require an acidic pH for absorption (itraconazole, ketoconazole, iron, etc.).
- Patients taking long-term should have adequate calcium and vitamin D intake. (Calcium citrate formulations are preferred.)
- Short-term side effects: headache, abdominal pain, diarrhea, constipation, nausea
- Long-term side effects: increased risk of osteoporosis or fracture, vitamin B_{12} deficiency, hypomagnesemia

ONDANSETRON

Brand Names
- Zofran, Zuplenz

Pharmacologic Class
- 5-HT$_3$ receptor antagonist

Mechanism of Action
- 5-HT$_3$-receptor antagonist which blocks serotonin peripherally on vagal nerve terminals and in the chemoreceptor trigger zone of the CNS.

Dosage Forms
- Oral (tablet, disintegrating tablet, film), injection solution (IM/IV)

Common Uses
- Prevention of post-operative nausea and vomiting, chemotherapy-induced nausea and vomiting, and radiation-induced nausea and vomiting

Quick Facts
- May mask signs and symptoms of bowel obstruction following abdominal surgery or chemotherapy-induced nausea and vomiting.
- Serotonin syndrome may occur when medication is used by itself or concomitantly with other serotonergic medications.
- Do not remove disintegrating tablet or film from packaging until immediately before use.
- May cause QT prolongation.
- Side effects: headache, constipation, diarrhea, fatigue

OSELTAMIVIR

Brand Name
- Tamiflu

Pharmacologic Class
- Neuraminidase inhibitor

Mechanism of Action
- Inhibits the activity of influenza virus neuraminidase, which prevents the release of viral particles.

Dosage Forms
- Oral (capsule, powder for suspension)

Common Uses
- Prophylaxis and treatment of influenza (types A and B)

Quick Facts
- Treatment of influenza for patients who have been symptomatic for no more than 48 hours.
- Administer with food to decrease gastric irritation.
- Avoid administration of intranasal live attenuated influenza vaccine (LAIV) within 2 weeks before or 48 hours after oseltamivir use.
- Patients should be counseled to report signs of neuropsychiatric events, including abnormal behavior, delirium, or hallucinations.
- Side effects: diarrhea, nausea, vomiting, headache, insomnia

OXCARBAZEPINE

Brand Name
- Trileptal

Pharmacologic Class
- Anticonvulsant

Mechanism of Action
- Mechanism of action remains unknown. Oxcarbazepine may produce its anticonvulsant effect by blocking voltage-sensitive sodium channels, which stabilizes hyperexcited neural membranes, inhibits repetitive neuronal firing, and decreases the propagation of synaptic impulses.

Dosage Forms
- Oral (tablet, suspension)

Common Use
- Treatment of epilepsy (partial seizures)

Quick Facts
- Serious and sometimes fatal dermatologic reactions including toxic epidermal necrolysis and Stevens-Johnson syndrome can occur, especially in patients with the HLA-B*1502 gene who are almost exclusively of Asian ancestry.
- Approximately 25% to 30% of patients who have had hypersensitivity reactions to carbamazepine will experience hypersensitivity reactions with oxcarbazepine.
- Clinically significant hyponatremia may occur. Monitor serum sodium levels periodically, particularly during the first 3 months of therapy. Patients should report symptoms of low sodium, including nausea, fatigue, confusion, and headache.
- Administer extended-release tablets on an empty stomach, at least 1 hour before or 2 hours after a meal. Immediate-release dosage forms can be taken without regard to meals.
- Potent CYP3A4 inducer.
- Side effects: fatigue, ataxia, diplopia, abdominal pain

OXYBUTYNIN

Brand Names
- Ditropan XL, Oxytrol, Gelnique

Pharmacologic Class
- Anticholinergic

Mechanism of Action
- Inhibits the muscarinic action of acetylcholine on smooth muscle, which causes bladder smooth muscle relaxation.

Dosage Forms
- Oral (tablet, syrup), transdermal (gel, patch)

Common Use
- Treatment of overactive bladder

Quick Facts
- Contraindicated in patients with uncontrolled narrow-angle glaucoma, urinary retention, or gastric retention.
- Medication may cause heat prostration when used in a hot environment due to decreased sweating.
- Increased drowsiness may occur with concomitant alcohol use.
- Transdermal forms cause less dry mouth and constipation than oral forms.
- Side effects: dry mouth, blurred vision, urinary retention, constipation

OXYCODONE

Brand Names
- OxyCONTIN, Roxicodone, Xtampza ER

Pharmacologic Class
- Opioid analgesic

Mechanism of Action
- Binds to the mu opioid receptor, which reduces neuronal cell excitability and transmission of nociceptive impulses.

Dosage Forms
- Oral (tablet, capsule, solution)

Common Use
- Treatment of moderate to severe pain

Quick Facts
- DEA Schedule II
- Black Box Warnings – Serious, life-threatening, or fatal respiratory depression may occur. Concomitant use with benzodiazepines increases risk of sedation, respiratory depression, coma, or death. Concomitant use with CYP3A4 inhibitors, or discontinuation of CYP3A4 inducers, can result in a fatal overdose of oxycodone. Prolonged use of oxycodone during pregnancy can result in neonatal opioid withdrawal syndrome.
- Extended-release oxycodone is for use only in opioid-tolerant patients for the management of persistent, moderate to severe chronic pain that requires continuous, around-the-clock opioid administration for an extended period of time.
- Do not break, chew, or crush long-acting forms.
- Side effects: somnolence, constipation, pruritus, sweating, dry mouth

PANTOPRAZOLE

Brand Name
- Protonix

Pharmacologic Class
- PPI

Mechanism of Action
- Suppresses gastric acid secretion by inhibiting the H^+/K^+-ATPase pump in parietal cells, blocking the final step of acid production.

Dosage Forms
- Oral (tablet, packet), intravenous (powder for solution)

Common Uses
- Treatment of GERD, erosive esophagitis, and Zollinger-Ellison syndrome

Quick Facts
- Take at least 30 to 60 minutes before eating.
- Do not abruptly discontinue. Medication should be tapered to avoid acid rebound.
- Use with caution with other medications that require an acidic pH for absorption (itraconazole, ketoconazole, iron, etc.).
- Patients taking long-term should have adequate calcium and vitamin D intake (calcium citrate formulations will have improved absorption in basic pH).
- Short-term side effects: headache, dizziness, diarrhea, constipation, abdominal pain
- Long-term side effects: increased risk of osteoporosis or fracture, vitamin B_{12} deficiency, hypomagnesemia

PAROXETINE

Brand Name
- Paxil

Pharmacologic Class
- SSRI

Mechanism of Action
- Inhibits the reuptake of serotonin in presynaptic neurons of the CNS.

Dosage Forms
- Oral (tablet, suspension)

Common Uses
- Treatment of depression, obsessive-compulsive disorder, panic disorder, premenstrual dysphoric disorder, post-traumatic stress disorder, and hot flashes due to menopause

Quick Facts
- Black Box Warning – Increased risk of suicidal thoughts and behavior in children, adolescents, and young adults.
- Potent CYP2D6 inhibitor.
- Associated with more weight gain than other SSRIs.
- May increase the risk of bleeding events. Concomitant use of aspirin, NSAIDs, warfarin, and other anticoagulants can increase risk.
- Do not abruptly discontinue medication.
- Use is contraindicated during or within 14 days of MAOI administration.
- Patients should report symptoms of hyponatremia, including headache, confusion, and weakness.
- Side effects: somnolence, insomnia, dry mouth, nausea

PENICILLIN V POTASSIUM

Brand Names
- Veetids, Pen VK

Pharmacologic Class
- Penicillin antibiotic

Mechanism of Action
- Inhibits bacterial cell wall synthesis by binding to one or more of the penicillin-binding proteins, which inhibits the final transpeptidation step of peptidoglycan synthesis in bacterial cell walls.

Dosage Forms
- Oral (tablet, powder for solution)

Common Uses
- Treatment of upper respiratory tract infections, otitis media, and skin and soft tissue infections; prophylaxis of bacterial endocarditis and rheumatic fever

Quick Facts
- Administer at even intervals to minimize variation in peak and trough serum levels.
- Preferably taken on an empty stomach 1 hour before or 2 hours after meals with a full glass of water to increase absorption.
- Store reconstituted oral solution in refrigerator.
- Side effects: diarrhea, nausea, vomiting, rash, black hairy tongue

PHENTERMINE

Brand Names
- Adipex-P, Lomaira

Pharmacologic Class
- CNS stimulant and anorexiant

Mechanism of Action
- Sympathomimetic amine that increases norepineph-rine release in the CNS, which suppresses appetite.

Dosage Forms
- Oral (tablet, capsule)

Common Use
- Treatment of obesity

Quick Facts
- DEA Schedule IV
- For use only in patients with a BMI ≥ 30 or ≥ 27 in the presence of other risk factors (e.g., diabetes, hyper-lipidemia, controlled hypertension).
- Contraindicated with concomitant use or use within 14 days of MAOI administration. Also contraindicated with cardiovascular disease (e.g., coronary artery dis-ease, arrhythmias, stroke, congestive heart failure, un-controlled hypertension).
- Do not administer in the evening due to the risk of insomnia.
- Rare cases of primary pulmonary hypertension have been reported.
- Side effects: dry mouth, taste disturbances, tremor, dizziness

PHENYTOIN

Brand Names
- Dilantin, Phenytek

Pharmacologic Class
- Anticonvulsant

Mechanism of Action
- Stabilizes neuronal membranes by possibly increasing efflux of sodium ions across cell membranes in the motor cortex during generation of nerve impulses.

Dosage Forms
- Oral (capsule, chewable tablet, suspension), injection (solution)

Common Use
- Treatment of epilepsy (partial and generalized onset seizures and status epilepticus)

Quick Facts
- Black Box Warning (injection only) – Maximum IV infusion rate should not exceed 50 mg/min because of the risk of severe hypotension and cardiac arrhythmias.
- Serious and sometimes fatal dermatologic reactions including toxic epidermal necrolysis and Stevens-Johnson syndrome can occur, especially in patients with the HLA-B*1502 gene who are almost exclusively of Asian ancestry.
- Injection should be mixed in normal saline only.
- Enteral tube feedings decrease phenytoin absorption. Feeds should be held 1 to 2 hours before and after phenytoin administration.
- May cause gingival hyperplasia. Patients should practice good dental hygiene.
- Potent CYP450 inducer.
- Side effects: drowsiness, osteoporosis, skin thickening of facial features, hirsutism

PIOGLITAZONE

Brand Name
▪ Actos

Pharmacologic Class
▪ Thiazolidinedione

Mechanism of Action
▪ Agonist at peroxisome proliferator-activated receptor-gamma, which regulates the transcription of genes involved in the control of glucose and lipid metabolism in skeletal muscle, adipose tissue, and the liver.

Dosage Form
▪ Oral (tablet)

Common Use
▪ Treatment of type 2 diabetes

Quick Facts
▪ Black Box Warning – May cause or worsen heart failure. Use is not recommended in patients with symptomatic heart failure and is contraindicated in patients with NYHA Class III or IV heart failure.
▪ Medication is dependent on the presence of insulin for its mechanism of action. (Do not use in type 1 diabetics or for the treatment of diabetic ketoacidosis.)
▪ Use is not recommended in patients with active bladder cancer.
▪ Monitor LFTs prior to initiation of therapy and periodically thereafter.
▪ Side effects: edema, upper respiratory tract infection, headache, myalgia

POLYETHYLENE GLYCOL

Brand Names
- Miralax, Glycolax

Pharmacologic Class
- Laxative

Mechanism of Action
- Osmotic agent which causes water to be retained in the stool.

Dosage Form
- Oral (powder for solution)

Common Use
- Treatment of constipation

Quick Facts
- Contraindicated in patients with a bowel obstruction.
- Symptomatic improvement may not be seen for 2 to 4 days. Medication should not be used for more than 2 weeks unless approved by healthcare provider.
- Mix powder with 4 to 8 oz. of water, juice, soda, coffee, or tea prior to administration.
- Side effects: nausea, abdominal bloating, cramping, diarrhea, flatulence

POTASSIUM CHLORIDE

Brand Names
- K-Dur, Klor-Con

Pharmacologic Class
- Electrolyte supplement

Mechanism of Action
- Potassium is the principal intracellular cation of most body tissues and is essential for several physiological processes, including the maintenance of intracellular tonicity, the transmission of nerve impulses, the contraction of cardiac, skeletal, and smooth muscle, and the maintenance of normal renal function.

Dosage Forms
- Oral (tablet, capsule, solution, powder for solution), intravenous (solution)

Common Uses
- Treatment and prevention of hypokalemia

Quick Facts
- Normal adult plasma concentration of potassium is 3.5 to 5 mEq/L.
- Administer oral forms with food and a full glass of water to prevent gastric irritation.
- Potassium must be diluted prior to parenteral administration and should not be given IV push.
- Concomitant use with potassium-sparing diuretics, aldosterone antagonists, ACEIs, or salt substitutes containing potassium may cause hyperkalemia.
- Slow release potassium tablets and capsules should be reserved for patients who cannot tolerate or have compliance problems with liquid or effervescent dosage forms due to the risk of intestinal and gastric ulceration and bleeding.
- Side effects: vomiting, flatulence, abdominal pain, diarrhea

PRAMIPEXOLE

Brand Name
- Mirapex

Pharmacologic Class
- Dopamine agonist

Mechanism of Action
- Mechanism of action is believed to be related to its ability to stimulate dopamine receptors in the striatum.

Dosage Form
- Oral (tablet)

Common Uses
- Treatment of Parkinson's disease and restless legs syndrome (immediate release only)

Quick Facts
- Reduce dosage in renal impairment (CrCl < 50 mL/min).
- Patients should report a new onset or exacerbation of dyskinesia.
- Take medication with food to decrease nausea.
- Do not abruptly discontinue medication.
- Avoid alcohol and other CNS depressants.
- Side effects: drowsiness, sleep attacks, dizziness, nausea, orthostatic hypotension, hallucinations

PRASUGREL

Brand Name
- Effient

Pharmacologic Class
- $P2Y_{12}$ antagonist

Mechanism of Action
- Inhibits the binding of ADP to its platelet $P2Y_{12}$ receptor, which prevents activation of the GPIIb/IIIa complex and platelet aggregation.

Dosage Form
- Oral (tablet)

Common Uses
- Reduction of thrombotic events in patients with acute coronary syndrome who are to be managed with PCI for unstable angina, non-ST-elevation MI, or ST-elevation MI

Quick Facts
- Black Box Warnings – Can cause significant and sometimes fatal bleeding and should not be used in patients with active pathological bleeding or with a history of TIA or stroke. Prasugrel is generally not recommended in patients ≥ 75 years old. Do not start prasugrel in patients likely to undergo urgent CABG surgery, and discontinue at least 7 days prior to any surgery. Additional risk factors for bleeding include body weight < 60 kg, a tendency to experience bleeding, and concomitant use of medications that increase the risk of bleeding.
- Rare cases of thrombotic thrombocytopenia purpura (TTP) have been reported. Symptoms include fever, fatigue, purplish bruises, and yellowing of the skin or eyes.
- Side effects: bleeding, bruising, hyperlipidemia, headache, back pain

PRAVASTATIN

Brand Name
- Pravachol

Pharmacologic Class
- HMG-CoA reductase inhibitor

Mechanism of Action
- Inhibits HMG-CoA reductase, preventing the conversion of HMG-CoA to mevalonate (the rate-limiting step in cholesterol synthesis).

Dosage Form
- Oral (tablet)

Common Use
- Treatment of hyperlipidemia

Quick Facts
- CYP3A4 inhibitors can increase plasma concentration.
- Contraindicated in active liver disease and in pregnancy and lactation.
- Monitor LFTs at baseline and periodically thereafter.
- Patients taking cholestyramine or colestipol concomitantly should take pravastatin at least 1 hour before or 4 hours after these medications.
- Limit alcohol intake.
- Can be taken at any time of day.
- Side effects: diarrhea, arthralgia, myalgia, increased liver enzymes, upper respiratory tract infection

PREDNISOLONE (oral)

Brand Names
- Orapred, Millipred

Pharmacologic Class
- Corticosteroid

Mechanism of Action
- Binds to cytoplasmic receptors in cells. The steroid-receptor complex then enters the nucleus of cells where it modifies transcription and thus the synthesis of proteins and enzymes involved with inflammation.

Dosage Forms
- Oral (tablet, solution, syrup)

Common Uses
- Treatment of various allergic and inflammatory diseases (endocrine disorders, respiratory diseases, rheumatic disorders, etc.)

Quick Facts
- Patients on long-term therapy should avoid live or live-attenuated vaccines due to drug-induced immunosuppression.
- Take with food to decrease GI upset.
- Contraindicated in patients with systemic fungal infections because the infections may be exacerbated.
- Taper dose to prevent withdrawal symptoms if used longer than 2 weeks.
- Storage requirements for oral solution vary by manufacturer.
- Short-term side effects: insomnia, stomach upset, fluid retention, increased appetite
- Long-term side effects: Cushing's syndrome, osteoporosis, muscle wasting, growth suppression in children

PREDNISONE

Brand Names
▪ Deltasone, Rayos

Pharmacologic Class
▪ Corticosteroid

Mechanism of Action
▪ Binds to cytoplasmic receptors in cells. The steroid-receptor complex then enters the nucleus of cells where it modifies transcription and thus the synthesis of proteins and enzymes involved with inflammation.

Dosage Forms
▪ Oral (tablet, solution)

Common Uses
▪ Treatment of various allergic and inflammatory diseases (endocrine disorders, respiratory diseases, rheumatic disorders, etc.)

Quick Facts
▪ Patients on long-term therapy should avoid live or live-attenuated vaccines due to drug-induced immunosuppression.
▪ Take with food to decrease GI upset.
▪ Contraindicated in patients with systemic fungal infections because the infections may be exacerbated.
▪ Taper dose to prevent withdrawal symptoms if used longer than 2 weeks.
▪ Short-term side effects: insomnia, stomach upset, fluid retention, increased appetite
▪ Long-term side effects: Cushing's syndrome, osteoporosis, muscle wasting, growth suppression in children

PREGABALIN

Brand Name
- Lyrica

Pharmacologic Class
- Anticonvulsant

Mechanism of Action
- Binds to the alpha$_2$-delta subunit of voltage-gated calcium channels in the CNS, reducing the calcium-dependent release of excitatory neurotransmitters including glutamate, norepinephrine, serotonin, dopamine, substance P, and calcitonin gene-related peptide.

Dosage Forms
- Oral (tablet, capsule, solution)

Common Uses
- Treatment of fibromyalgia, neuropathic pain associated with diabetes or spinal cord injury, postherpetic neuralgia, and partial seizures

Quick Facts
- DEA Schedule V
- May cause peripheral edema. Use caution when using concomitantly with thiazolidinediones.
- May cause myopathy. Patients should report muscle pain, tenderness, or weakness.
- Avoid abrupt discontinuation. Taper gradually over 1 week.
- Avoid alcohol and other CNS depressants.
- Side effects: weight gain, blurred vision, dry mouth, constipation, somnolence

PROCHLORPERAZINE

Brand Names
- Compazine, Compro

Pharmacologic Class
- Antipsychotic and antiemetic

Mechanism of Action
- Inhibits dopamine D_1 and D_2 receptors in the brain, including the chemoreceptor trigger zone of the CNS. It can also block histaminergic, cholinergic, and noradrenergic receptors.

Dosage Forms
- Oral (tablet), injection solution (IM/IV), rectal (suppository)

Common Uses
- Treatment of severe nausea and vomiting

Quick Facts
- Black Box Warning – Increased risk of mortality in elderly patients with dementia-related psychosis.
- May cause QT prolongation.
- Contraindicated in children < 2 years old or under 20 pounds.
- Medication may impair heat regulation. Patients should use caution with activities leading to increased core temperature, including strenuous exercise, dehydration, etc.
- Patients should report symptoms of tardive dyskinesia or neuroleptic malignant syndrome.
- Side effects: dizziness, blurred vision, drowsiness, skin reactions

PROGESTERONE

Brand Names
- Prometrium, Crinone, Endometrin

Pharmacologic Class
- Progestin

Mechanism of Action
- Converts a proliferative endometrium into a secretory one, reducing endometrial growth. Also inhibits the secretion of pituitary gonadotropins, which prevents follicular maturation and ovulation.

Dosage Forms
- Oral (capsule), vaginal (gel, tablet), intramuscular (oil)

Common Uses
- Prevention of endometrial hyperplasia (oral); treatment of amenorrhea (IM) and infertility (vaginal gel, tablet)

Quick Facts
- Black Box Warnings (oral use) – Estrogen plus progestins should not be used for the prevention of cardiovascular disease. Increased risks of MI, stroke, invasive breast cancer, pulmonary emboli, and DVT in postmenopausal women (50 to 79 years of age) using estrogens combined with progestins have been reported. An increased risk of developing probable dementia in postmenopausal women ≥ 65 years old has been reported when using estrogen plus progestin.
- Oral capsules contain peanut oil and are contraindicated in patients with a peanut allergy.
- When using vaginal form, patient should avoid using other vaginal drugs 6 hours before or 6 hours after using progesterone.
- Side effects: breast pain, headache, dizziness, joint pain

PROMETHAZINE

Brand Names
- Phenergan, Promethegan, Phenadoz

Pharmacologic Class
- H_1 antagonist

Mechanism of Action
- Competitively inhibits histamine at H_1 receptor sites.

Dosage Forms
- Oral (tablet, syrup, solution), injection solution (IM/IV), rectal (suppository)

Common Uses
- Prevention of nausea and vomiting; treatment of allergic conditions

Quick Facts
- Black Box Warnings – Should not be used in children < 2 years old due to the risk of fatal respiratory depression. Injection solution can cause severe tissue injury (including gangrene) regardless of the route of administration. Deep IM injection is the preferred route of administration due to the risks of IV administration. Subcutaneous injection is contraindicated.
- May cause QT prolongation.
- Patients should report symptoms of tardive dyskinesia or neuroleptic malignant syndrome.
- Side effects: drowsiness, dry mouth, blurred vision, rash

PROPAFENONE

Brand Name
- Rythmol

Pharmacologic Class
- Antiarrhythmic (Class Ic)

Mechanism of Action
- Blocks sodium channels to restrict the entry of sodium into the cardiac muscle cells, causing a decrease in excitability of the cells. Propafenone also has local anesthetic effects and a direct stabilizing action on myocardial membranes.

Dosage Forms
- Oral (tablet, capsule)

Common Uses
- Treatment of ventricular arrhythmias and symptomatic atrial fibrillation in patients without structural heart disease

Quick Facts
- Black Box Warning – Propafenone has proarrhythmic potential and may induce or exacerbate cardiac arrhythmias in patients with structural heart disease. Given the lack of any evidence that these drugs improve survival, antiarrhythmic agents should generally be avoided in patients with non-life-threatening ventricular arrhythmias, even if the patients are experiencing unpleasant, but not life-threatening, symptoms or signs.
- Contraindications include AV block, bradycardia, cardiogenic shock, bronchospastic disorders, and severe obstructive pulmonary disease.
- Major CYP2D6 substrate.
- Side effects: dizziness, palpitations, chest pain, edema, taste disturbance

PROPRANOLOL

Brand Names
- Inderal XL/LA, InnoPran XL

Pharmacologic Class
- Beta$_1$/beta$_2$-blocker

Mechanism of Action
- Blocks stimulation of beta$_1$ (myocardial) and beta$_2$ (pulmonary, vascular)-adrenergic receptors which reduces cardiac output, reduces exercise-induced tachycardia and/or isoproterenol-induced tachycardia, and reduces reflex orthostatic tachycardia.

Dosage Forms
- Oral (tablet, capsule, solution), intravenous (solution)

Common Uses
- Treatment of hypertension, angina pectoris (chronic), essential tremor, migraine prevention, and MI (early treatment and secondary prevention)

Quick Facts
- Black Box Warning – Abrupt cessation may precipitate angina, MI, arrhythmias, or rebound hypertension.
- Contraindications include bronchial asthma or related bronchial spastic condition, 2nd or 3rd degree AV block (if no pacemaker is present), cardiogenic shock, and severe sinus bradycardia.
- Infuse IV form at a rate of 1 mg/minute.
- Extended-release capsules can be taken with or without food but must be consistent. Immediate-release tablets should be taken with food.
- Side effects: diarrhea, dizziness, vomiting, fatigue

QUETIAPINE

Brand Name
- Seroquel

Pharmacologic Class
- Antipsychotic

Mechanism of Action
- Blocks dopamine D_2 and serotonin 5-HT_{2A} receptors. Also blocks histamine H_1 and alpha$_1$- and alpha$_2$-adrenergic receptors.

Dosage Form
- Oral (tablet)

Common Uses
- Treatment of bipolar disorder, major depressive disorder, and schizophrenia

Quick Facts
- Black Box Warnings – Elderly patients with dementia-related psychosis treated with antipsychotic drugs are at an increased risk of death. There is an increased risk of suicidal thoughts and behavior in children, adolescents, and young adults.
- Can prolong the QT interval.
- Patients should be counseled to report signs of extrapyramidal symptoms (restlessness, tremor, stiffness, etc.) or neuroleptic malignant syndrome (sweating, fever, muscle rigidity, etc.).
- Monitor for hyperglycemia, dyslipidemia, and weight gain.
- An eye exam for cataracts is recommended when beginning therapy and every 6 months thereafter.
- Side effects: somnolence, orthostatic hypotension, constipation, dizziness, dry mouth

QUINAPRIL

Brand Name
- Accupril

Pharmacologic Class
- ACE inhibitor

Mechanism of Action
- Inhibits the angiotensin converting enzyme (ACE), which prevents the conversion of angiotensin I to angiotensin II, a potent vasoconstrictor.

Dosage Form
- Oral (tablet)

Common Uses
- Treatment of hypertension and heart failure

Quick Facts
- Black Box Warning – Discontinue use as soon as possible if pregnancy is detected.
- Contraindicated in patients with a history of angioedema, concomitant use with aliskiren in diabetic patients, concomitant use with neprilysin inhibitor, or within 36 hours of switching to or from a neprilysin inhibitor.
- Use caution in patients with impaired renal function.
- Patients should avoid potassium supplements or salt substitutes containing potassium without first consulting healthcare provider.
- Side effects: cough, dizziness, headache, fatigue, angioedema

RALOXIFENE

Brand Name
- Evista

Pharmacologic Class
- SERM

Mechanism of Action
- Selective estrogen receptor modulator that acts as an estrogen agonist in bone to decrease bone resorption and bone turnover. Also acts as an estrogen antagonist in uterine and breast tissues.

Dosage Form
- Oral (tablet)

Common Uses
- Treatment and prevention of osteoporosis in postmenopausal women; prevention of invasive breast cancer in postmenopausal women

Quick Facts
- Black Box Warning – Increased risk of DVT and PE, increased risk of death due to stroke in postmenopausal women with coronary heart disease or at increased risk for major coronary events.
- Contraindicated in women with active or history of venous thromboembolic events.
- Medication should be discontinued at least 72 hours prior to and during prolonged immobilization (post-surgical recovery, prolonged bed rest, etc.) and prolonged restrictions of movement during travel should be avoided to decrease the risk of thromboembolic events.
- Cholestyramine reduces the bioavailability of raloxifene and concurrent use is not recommended.
- Side effects: hot flashes, weight gain, leg cramps, peripheral edema

RAMIPRIL

Brand Name
- Altace

Pharmacologic Class
- ACE inhibitor

Mechanism of Action
- Inhibits the angiotensin converting enzyme (ACE), which prevents the conversion of angiotensin I to angiotensin II, a potent vasoconstrictor.

Dosage Form
- Oral (capsule)

Common Uses
- Treatment of hypertension and heart failure in post-MI patients; reduction in risk of MI, stroke, and death from cardiovascular causes

Quick Facts
- Black Box Warning – Discontinue use as soon as possible if pregnancy is detected.
- Contraindicated in patients with a history of angi-oedema, concomitant use with aliskiren in diabetic patients, concomitant use with neprilysin inhibitor, or within 36 hours of switching to or from a nepri-lysin inhibitor.
- Use caution in patients with impaired renal function.
- Patients should avoid potassium supplements or salt substitutes containing potassium without first consulting healthcare provider.
- Side effects: cough, dizziness, headache, hypoten-sion, fatigue

RANOLAZINE

Brand Name
- Ranexa

Pharmacologic Class
- Antianginal agent

Mechanism of Action
- Mechanism of antianginal effect is unknown. Ranolazine inhibits the late phase inward sodium current in cardiac myocytes, which reduces intracellular sodium levels and calcium influx via Na^+-Ca^{2+} exchange.

Dosage Form
- Oral (tablet)

Common Use
- Treatment of chronic angina

Quick Facts
- Contraindicated with strong CYP3A4 inhibitors and CYP3A4 inducers.
- Maximum dose of ranolazine is 500 mg twice daily when used concomitantly with moderate CYP3A4 inhibitors.
- Avoid grapefruit and grapefruit juice while taking medication.
- May cause QT prolongation.
- Side effects: dizziness, headache, nausea, constipation

RIFAXIMIN

Brand Name
- Xifaxan

Pharmacologic Class
- Rifamycin antibiotic

Mechanism of Action
- Inhibits RNA synthesis by binding to RNA polymerase.

Dosage Form
- Oral (tablet)

Common Uses
- Treatment of traveler's diarrhea and irritable bowel syndrome with diarrhea; prophylaxis of hepatic encephalopathy recurrence

Quick Facts
- Rifaximin has minimal systemic absorption and is not effective for the treatment of other types of infections.
- Patients with traveler's diarrhea should report if symptoms get worse or persist after 24 to 48 hours of therapy.
- Patients with hepatic encephalopathy should report symptoms of *C. difficile*-associated diarrhea during or after therapy.
- Side effects: nausea, vomiting, headache, peripheral edema

RISEDRONATE

Brand Names
- Actonel, Atelvia

Pharmacologic Class
- Bisphosphonate

Mechanism of Action
- Inhibits osteoclast-mediated bone resorption.

Dosage Form
- Oral (tablet)

Common Uses
- Treatment and prevention of osteoporosis; treatment of Paget's disease

Quick Facts
- Immediate-release tablet should be taken in the morning with 6 to 8 oz. of plain water at least 30 minutes before the first food, beverage, and other medications of the day.
- Delayed-release tablet should be taken in the morning immediately after breakfast with at least 4 oz. of plain water.
- Patient should stay upright for at least 30 minutes after administration to prevent esophageal irritation.
- Products containing calcium, iron, magnesium, or aluminum should be taken at a separate time. Concomitant use of PPIs and H_2 blockers and delayed-release tablets is not recommended.
- Side effects: abdominal pain, acid regurgitation, constipation, diarrhea, esophagitis
- Less common side effects: atypical femur fracture, osteonecrosis of the jaw

RISPERIDONE

Brand Name
- Risperdal

Pharmacologic Class
- Antipsychotic

Mechanism of Action
- Blocks dopamine D_2 and serotonin $5\text{-}HT_{2A}$ receptors. Also blocks histamine H_1 and $alpha_1$- and $alpha_2$-adrenergic receptors.

Dosage Forms
- Oral (tablet, disintegrating tablet, solution), intramuscular (powder for injection), subcutaneous (powder for injection)

Common Uses
- Treatment of bipolar disorder, schizophrenia, and irritability associated with autistic disorder

Quick Facts
- Black Box Warning – Elderly patients with dementia-related psychosis treated with antipsychotics are at an increased risk of death compared to placebo. Most deaths appeared to be either cardiovascular (e.g., heart failure, sudden death) or infectious (e.g., pneumonia) in nature.
- Can prolong the QT interval.
- Patients should be counseled to report signs of extrapyramidal symptoms, tardive dyskinesia (restlessness, tremor, stiffness, etc.) or neuroleptic malignant syndrome (sweating, fever, muscle rigidity, etc.).
- Monitor for hyperglycemia, dyslipidemia, and weight gain.
- May cause hyperprolactinemia.
- Side effects: parkinsonism, insomnia, anxiety, somnolence

RIVAROXABAN

Brand Name
- Xarelto

Pharmacologic Class
- Factor Xa inhibitor

Mechanism of Action
- Competitively inhibits free and clot-bound factor Xa, resulting in decreased thrombin generation and thrombus formation.

Dosage Form
- Oral (tablet)

Common Uses
- Treatment and prophylaxis of DVT or PE; used to reduce the risk of stroke and systemic embolism in patients with nonvalvular atrial fibrillation (AF), and used to reduce the risk of major cardiovascular events in patients with chronic coronary artery disease or peripheral artery disease; prophylaxis of DVT in patients who have undergone hip or knee replacement surgery, and prophylaxis of venous thromboembolism (VTE) in acutely ill medical patients

Quick Facts
- Black Box Warnings – Premature discontinuation increases the risk of thrombotic events. To reduce risk consider coverage with another anticoagulant if rivaroxaban is discontinued for a reason other than pathological bleeding or completion of therapy. Patients undergoing neuroaxial anesthesia or spinal puncture have an increased risk of epidural or spinal hematomas which could result in permanent paralysis.
- 15 and 20 mg tablets should be administered with food.
- Side effects: bleeding, syncope, pruritis, muscle spasms, extremity pain

ROPINIROLE

Brand Name
- Requip

Pharmacologic Class
- Dopamine agonist

Mechanism of Action
- Agonist at both D_2 and D_3 dopamine receptors. Its mechanism of action is believed to be due to stimulation of postsynaptic dopamine D_2 receptors within the caudate-putamen in the brain.

Dosage Form
- Oral (tablet)

Common Uses
- Treatment of Parkinson's disease and restless leg syndrome (immediate release only)

Quick Facts
- Cigarette smoking increases clearance of medication. Patients should inform their prescriber if they plan to start or stop smoking.
- Patients should report a new onset or exacerbation of dyskinesia.
- Take medication with food to decrease nausea.
- Do not abruptly discontinue medication.
- Avoid alcohol and other CNS depressants.
- Side effects: drowsiness, sleep attacks, nausea, dizziness, orthostatic hypotension, hallucinations

ROSUVASTATIN

Brand Names
- Crestor, Ezallor

Pharmacologic Class
- HMG-CoA reductase inhibitor

Mechanism of Action
- Inhibits HMG-CoA reductase, preventing the conversion of HMG-CoA to mevalonate (the rate-limiting step in cholesterol synthesis).

Dosage Forms
- Oral (tablet, capsule)

Common Use
- Treatment of hyperlipidemia

Quick Facts
- CYP3A4 inhibitors can increase plasma concentration.
- Contraindicated in active liver disease and in pregnancy and lactation.
- Monitor LFTs at baseline and periodically thereafter.
- Limit alcohol intake.
- Patients should not use aluminum or magnesium-containing antacids for at least 2 hours after taking medication.
- Can be taken at any time of day.
- Side effects: abdominal pain, myalgia, nausea, constipation

SAXAGLIPTAN

Brand Name
- Onglyza

Pharmacologic Class
- DPP-4 inhibitor

Mechanism of Action
- Prevents the dipeptidyl peptidase-4 (DPP-4) enzyme from degrading the incretin hormones glucagon-like peptide-1 (GLP-1) and glucose-dependent insulino-tropic polypeptide (GIP). These hormones increase insulin release and decrease glucagon levels.

Dosage Form
- Oral (tablet)

Common Use
- Treatment of type 2 diabetes

Quick Facts
- Recommended daily dose is 2.5 mg when medication is used in combination with strong CYP3A4 inhibitors, including ketoconazole, clarithromycin, etc.
- Reduce dosage in renal impairment (eGFR < 45 mL/min/1.73m^2).
- Patients should be counseled to report symptoms of congestive heart failure, acute pancreatitis, and bullous pemphigoid.
- Side effects: peripheral edema, headache, upper respiratory tract infection, urinary tract infection

SERTRALINE

Brand Name
- Zoloft

Pharmacologic Class
- SSRI

Mechanism of Action
- Inhibits the reuptake of serotonin in presynaptic neurons of the CNS.

Dosage Forms
- Oral (tablet, solution)

Common Uses
- Treatment of depression, obsessive-compulsive disorder, panic disorder, post-traumatic stress disorder, social anxiety disorder, and premenstrual dysphoric disorder

Quick Facts
- Black Box Warning – Increased risk of suicidal thoughts and behavior in children, adolescents, and young adults.
- Risk of QT interval prolongation.
- May increase the risk of bleeding events. Concomitant use of aspirin, NSAIDs, warfarin, and other anticoagulants can increase risk.
- Do not abruptly discontinue medication.
- Use is contraindicated during or within 14 days of MAOI administration.
- Patients should report symptoms of hyponatremia, including headache, confusion, and weakness.
- Side effects: somnolence, insomnia, headache, dyspepsia, nausea

SILDENAFIL

Brand Names
- Viagra, Revatio

Pharmacologic Class
- PDE-5 inhibitor

Mechanism of Action
- Inhibits phosphodiesterase-5, which increases levels of cyclic guanosine monophosphate (cGMP) within vascular smooth muscle cells, causing relaxation and vasodilation.

Dosage Forms
- Oral (tablet, powder for suspension), intravenous (solution)

Common Uses
- Treatment of erectile dysfunction and pulmonary arterial hypertension

Quick Facts
- Concomitant use with organic nitrates is contraindicated due to the risk of hypotension.
- Taking medication with a high fat meal slows absorption.
- For ED, take approximately 1 hour (30 minutes to 4 hours) before sexual activity.
- For pulmonary arterial hypertension, doses should be taken approximately 4 to 6 hours apart.
- Patients should be counseled to immediately report priapism, vision loss in one or both eyes, and sudden decrease or loss of hearing.
- Side effects: flushing, headache, abnormal vision, dyspepsia

SIMVASTATIN

Brand Name
- Zocor

Pharmacologic Class
- HMG-CoA reductase inhibitor

Mechanism of Action
- Inhibits HMG-CoA reductase, preventing the conversion of HMG-CoA to mevalonate (the rate-limiting step in cholesterol synthesis).

Dosage Forms
- Oral (tablet, suspension)

Common Use
- Treatment of hyperlipidemia

Quick Facts
- CYP3A4 inhibitors can increase plasma concentration.
- Contraindicated in active liver disease and in pregnancy and lactation.
- Monitor LFTs at baseline and periodically thereafter.
- Limit alcohol intake and avoid grapefruit and grapefruit juice.
- The 80 mg dose should only be used in patients who have already been taking simvastatin for 12 months without signs of muscle toxicity.
- Take in the evening for maximal efficacy.
- Side effects: constipation, myalgia, abdominal pain, upper respiratory tract infection

SITAGLIPTAN

Brand Name
- Januvia

Pharmacologic Class
- DPP-4 inhibitor

Mechanism of Action
- Prevents the dipeptidyl peptidase-4 (DPP-4) enzyme from degrading the incretin hormones glucagon-like peptide-1 (GLP-1) and glucose-dependent insulinotropic polypeptide (GIP). These hormones increase insulin release and decrease glucagon levels.

Dosage Form
- Oral (tablet)

Common Use
- Treatment of type 2 diabetes

Quick Facts
- Reduce dosage in renal impairment (eGFR < 45 mL/min/1.73m^2).
- Patients should be counseled to report symptoms of congestive heart failure, acute pancreatitis, and bullous pemphigoid.
- Side effects: upper respiratory tract infection, nasopharyngitis, headache

SODIUM FLUORIDE (topical)

Brand Names
- PreviDent, Clinpro 5000, DentaGel, Gel-Kam

Pharmacologic Class
- Fluoride supplement

Mechanism of Action
- Protects teeth from acid demineralization, strengthens tooth enamel, and prevents tooth decay by bacteria.

Dosage Forms
- Topical (cream, gel, paste, rinse)

Common Use
- Prevention of dental caries

Quick Facts
- Excessive doses may cause dental fluorosis (mottling of tooth enamel).
- Do not take calcium supplements, products containing calcium, or ingest foods high in calcium 2 hours before or after sodium fluoride administration due to a decrease in fluoride absorption.
- Adults patients should not eat, drink, or rinse for 30 minutes after using topical dosage forms.
- Pediatric patients should rinse mouth thoroughly after using topical dosage forms, and should be supervised to prevent swallowing.
- Side effects with excessive doses: dental fluorosis, tooth pitting

SOLIFENACIN

Brand Name
- Vesicare

Pharmacologic Class
- Anticholinergic agent

Mechanism of Action
- Inhibits the muscarinic action of acetylcholine on smooth muscle, which causes bladder smooth muscle relaxation.

Dosage Form
- Oral (tablet)

Common Use
- Treatment of overactive bladder

Quick Facts
- Contraindicated in patients with uncontrolled narrow-angle glaucoma, urinary retention, and gastric retention.
- Reduce dosage in renal impairment (CrCl < 30 mL/min) to a maximum of 5 mg/day.
- Medication may cause heat prostration when used in a hot environment due to decreased sweating.
- May be associated with QT prolongation.
- Side effects: dry mouth, blurred vision, urinary tract infection, constipation

SPIRONOLACTONE

Brand Names
- Aldactone, CaroSpir

Pharmacologic Class
- Aldosterone receptor antagonist and potassium-sparing diuretic

Mechanism of Action
- Competes with aldosterone for receptor sites in the distal convoluted tubules to increase sodium, chloride, and water excretion, and decrease the excretion of potassium.

Dosage Forms
- Oral (tablet, suspension)

Common Uses
- Treatment of heart failure with reduced ejection fraction, hypertension, edema associated with hepatic cirrhosis or nephrotic syndrome, and primary hyperaldosteronism (tablets only)

Quick Facts
- Contraindicated in patients with hyperkalemia, Addison's disease, and concomitant use of eplerenone.
- Administer in the morning because of increased diuresis.
- Medication can cause electrolyte imbalances, including hyperkalemia, hyponatremia, hypocalcemia, hypomagnesemia, and hypochloremic alkalosis. Monitor potassium levels within 1 week of initiation or titration, then monitor potassium and other electrolytes periodically thereafter.
- Patients should avoid potassium supplements and foods containing high levels of potassium, including salt substitutes.
- Can be taken with or without food but must be consistent.
- Side effects: gynecomastia, menstrual changes, hirsutism, diarrhea, nausea

SUCRALFATE

Brand Name
- Carafate

Pharmacologic Class
- Cytoprotective agent

Mechanism of Action
- Forms a complex by binding to positively charged proteins, which creates a coating that protects the gastric lining against peptic acid, pepsin, and bile salts.

Dosage Forms
- Oral (tablet, suspension)

Common Uses
- Treatment of active duodenal ulcers (≤ 8 weeks), and maintenance therapy for duodenal ulcers (tablets only)

Quick Facts
- Administer on an empty stomach 1 hour before or 2 hours after meals.
- Avoid taking antacids 30 minutes before or after sucralfate.
- Sucralfate can decrease the absorption of other medications. In general, separate administration of other medications and sucralfate by at least 2 hours.
- Sucralfate is an aluminum complex and may cause aluminum toxicity. Use with caution in patients on dialysis or with chronic renal failure.
- Side effects: constipation, indigestion, nausea

SULFAMETHOXAZOLE-TRIMETHOPRIM

Brand Names
- Bactrim, Septra, Sulfatrim

Pharmacologic Class
- Combination sulfonamide and folic acid inhibitor

Mechanism of Action
- Sulfamethoxazole inhibits dihydrofolic acid formation from para-aminobenzoic acid, which interferes with bacterial folic acid synthesis and growth. Trimethoprim interferes with the production of folic acid by inhibiting bacterial dihydrofolate reductase.

Dosage Forms
- Oral (tablet, suspension), intravenous (solution)

Common Uses
- Treatment of UTIs, acute otitis media, *Pneumocystis* pneumonia, acute exacerbation of chronic bronchitis, and traveler's diarrhea

Quick Facts
- Contraindications include megaloblastic anemia due to folate deficiency.
- Use with caution during pregnancy due to the risk of congenital malformations.
- Administer with at least 8 oz. of water to prevent crystalluria.
- Side effects: nausea, vomiting, rash, photosensitivity

SULFASALAZINE

Brand Names
- Azulfidine, Sulfazine

Pharmacologic Class
- Aminosalicylate

Mechanism of Action
- Sulfasalazine is metabolized to its active components, sulfapyridine and mesalamine (5-ASA), by bacteria in the colon. The beneficial effects result primarily from mesalamine, which may block cyclooxygenase and inhibit prostaglandin formation in the colon. The mechanism of action of sulfasalazine and its metabolites in rheumatoid arthritis is unknown.

Dosage Forms
- Oral (tablet, delayed release tablet)

Common Uses
- Treatment of ulcerative colitis and rheumatoid arthritis

Quick Facts
- Contraindicated in patients with a hypersensitivity to sulfonamides or salicylates, and intestinal or urinary obstruction and porphyria.
- Medication should be administered in evenly divided doses after meals. Patients should maintain adequate hydration during therapy to prevent crystalluria.
- Medication decreases folate absorption and some patients may require supplementation.
- Medication may cause photosensitivity. Patients should limit sunlight and UV light exposure.
- Side effects: rash, abdominal pain, headache, yellow-orange coloration of skin or urine

SUMATRIPTAN

Brand Names
- Imitrex, Onzetra Xsail, Tosymra

Pharmacologic Class
- Serotonin receptor agonist

Mechanism of Action
- Agonist of serotonin 5-HT$_{1B/1D}$ receptors on intracranial blood vessels and sensory nerves of the trigeminal system, which constricts cranial blood vessels and inhibits the release of pro-inflammatory neuropeptides.

Dosage Forms
- Oral (tablet), nasal (solution, powder) subcutaneous (solution)

Common Uses
- Treatment of migraine and cluster headaches (subcutaneous dosage form)

Quick Facts
- Use is contraindicated during or within 14 days of MAO type A inhibitor discontinuation.
- Use is contraindicated within 24 hours of an ergotamine derivative or another 5-HT$_1$ agonist.
- Take at onset of migraine. When used orally, may repeat dose once in 2 hours if needed. When used nasally or subcutaneously, may repeat dose once in 1 hour if needed.
- Side effects: bad taste in mouth, throat or neck pressure, chest pain or tightness, dizziness

TACROLIMUS (systemic)

Brand Names
- Prograf, Astagraf XL, Envarsus XR

Pharmacologic Class
- Calcineurin inhibitor

Mechanism of Action
- Tacrolimus binds to an intracellular protein, FKBP-12, and forms a complex with calcineurin dependent proteins to inhibit calcineurin phosphatase activity. This inhibits T-lymphocyte activation and proliferation and T-helper-cell-dependent B-cell response.

Dosage Forms
- Oral (tablet, capsule, granules), intravenous (solution)

Common Uses
- Prophylaxis of organ rejection in renal, cardiac, and hepatic transplants

Quick Facts
- Black Box Warnings – Increased risk of developing lymphomas and other malignancies, particularly of the skin; increased risk of developing bacterial, viral, fungal, and protozoal infections, including opportunistic infections.
- Immediate-release dosage forms are not interchangeable with extended-release dosage forms.
- Immediate-release dosage forms can be taken with or without food but must be consistent.
- Extended-release dosage forms should be taken on an empty stomach 1 hour before or 2 hours after a meal.
- Avoid live vaccines during therapy.
- Avoid grapefruit and grapefruit juice. Avoid alcohol with extended-release dosage forms.
- Side effects: hyperglycemia, hypertension, edema, headache, tremor, alopecia

TADALAFIL

Brand Names
- Cialis, Adcirca

Pharmacologic Class
- PDE-5 inhibitor

Mechanism of Action
- Inhibits phosphodiesterase-5, which increases levels of cyclic guanosine monophosphate (cGMP) within vascular smooth muscle cells, causing relaxation and vasodilation.

Dosage Form
- Oral (tablet)

Common Uses
- Treatment of erectile dysfunction and BPH (Cialis only) and pulmonary arterial hypertension (Adcirca only)

Quick Facts
- Concomitant use with organic nitrates is contraindicated due to the risk of hypotension.
- When used on an as-needed basis, take at least 30 minutes before sexual activity. When used on a once-daily basis, take at approximately the same time every day.
- For pulmonary arterial hypertension, daily dose should be administered all at once and not divided throughout the day.
- Patients should be counseled to immediately report priapism, vision loss in one or both eyes, and sudden decrease or loss of hearing.
- Side effects: flushing, headache, abnormal vision, back pain

TAMOXIFEN

Brand Names
- Nolvadex, Soltamox

Pharmacologic Class
- SERM

Mechanism of Action
- Competitively inhibits estrogen binding to its receptors in breasts and other tissues, producing a nuclear complex that decreases DNA synthesis and inhibits estrogen effects.

Dosage Forms
- Oral (tablet, solution)

Common Uses
- Treatment of estrogen receptor-positive metastatic breast cancer in adults; used as an adjuvant in the treatment of early stage estrogen receptor-positive breast cancer in adults; used to reduce the risk of invasive breast cancer after surgery and radiation in adult women with ductal carcinoma in situ; used to reduce the incidence of breast cancer in adult females at high risk

Quick Facts
- Black Box Warning – Serious and life-threatening uterine malignancies, stroke, and PE have been associated with tamoxifen use in the risk reduction setting (women with ductal carcinoma in situ and women at high risk for breast cancer).
- Medication must be converted to its active metabolites by CYP2D6.
- Females of reproductive potential should use nonhormonal contraception to avoid pregnancy during therapy and for 2 months following the last dose.
- Periodic ocular tests should be performed during treatment.
- Side effects: hot flashes, rash, bone pain, edema

TAMSULOSIN

Brand Name
- Flomax

Pharmacologic Class
- Alpha$_1$-blocker

Mechanism of Action
- Antagonist of alpha$_{1A}$-adrenergic receptors in the prostate, which relaxes the smooth muscle of the prostate and bladder neck.

Dosage Form
- Oral (capsule)

Common Use
- Treatment of BPH

Quick Facts
- Administer medication 30 minutes after the same meal each day.
- Medication may cause orthostatic hypotension, especially with first dose or a dose increase. Patients should be counseled to rise slowly from a sitting or lying position.
- Medication should not be used in patients with planned cataract or glaucoma surgery due to the risk of intraoperative floppy iris syndrome (IFIS).
- Side effects: headache, dizziness, back pain, asthenia

TEMAZEPAM

Brand Name
- Restoril

Pharmacologic Class
- Benzodiazepine

Mechanism of Action
- Causes CNS depression by potentiating the effects of GABA (an inhibitory neurotransmitter).

Dosage Form
- Oral (capsule)

Common Use
- Treatment of insomnia

Quick Facts
- DEA Schedule IV
- Black Box Warning – Concomitant use with opioids increases risk of sedation, respiratory depression, coma, or death.
- Indicated for the short-term treatment of insomnia (7 to 10 days).
- Avoid alcohol and other CNS depressants while taking medication.
- Metabolized to inactive compounds, therefore it may be less harmful for elderly patients or patients with hepatic impairment.
- Side effects: drowsiness, dizziness, euphoria, confusion

TERAZOSIN

Brand Name
- Hytrin

Pharmacologic Class
- Alpha$_1$-blocker

Mechanism of Action
- Antagonist of alpha$_1$-adrenergic receptors, which decreases systemic vascular resistance and relaxes the smooth muscle of the prostate and bladder neck.

Dosage Form
- Oral (capsule)

Common Uses
- Treatment of hypertension and BPH

Quick Facts
- To avoid first-dose syncope, administer first dose at bedtime and do not exceed 1 mg. If medication is discontinued for several days or a patient misses several doses, therapy should be restarted using the initial dosing regimen.
- Do not abruptly discontinue medication, as it may cause rebound hypertension.
- Side effects: headache, dizziness, asthenia, orthostatic hypotension

TESTOSTERONE

Brand Names
- Androderm, AndroGel, Testim

Pharmacologic Class
- Androgen

Mechanism of Action
- Endogenous androgen responsible for normal growth and development of male sex organs.

Dosage Forms
- Oral (capsule, buccal patch), topical/transdermal (gel, solution, patch), intramuscular (solution), subcutaneous (implant)

Common Use
- Treatment of hypogonadism

Quick Facts
- Black Box Warning (for all topical agents) – Virilization has been reported in children who were secondarily exposed to testosterone topical agents. Children should avoid contact with unwashed or unclothed testosterone application sites.
- Contraindicated in men with prostate cancer or breast cancer.
- May increase the risk of MI and stroke.
- Monitoring parameters include LFTs, lipid panel, PSA, hemoglobin/hematocrit, and testosterone levels.
- Side effects: hypertension, BPH, gynecomastia, acne

THYROID USP

Brand Names
- Armour Thyroid, Nature-Throid, Westhroid

Pharmacologic Class
- Thyroid supplement

Mechanism of Action
- Thyroid USP is a mix of T_3 and T_4, which exert their physiological actions through control of DNA transcription and protein synthesis. This results in an increased metabolic rate, decreased TSH production by the pituitary gland, and effects on lipid and carbohydrate metabolism.

Dosage Form
- Oral (tablet)

Common Use
- Treatment of hypothyroidism

Quick Facts
- Black Box Warning – Medication should not be used for the treatment of obesity or for weight loss. High doses may produce serious or life-threatening toxic effects.
- Administer in the morning on an empty stomach, 30 to 60 minutes before breakfast.
- Do not administer within 4 to 5 hours of cholestyramine or colestipol.
- Side effects if dose is too high: palpitations, sweating, weight loss

TICAGRELOR

Brand Name
- Brilinta

Pharmacologic Class
- $P2Y_{12}$ inhibitor

Mechanism of Action
- Inhibits the binding of ADP to its platelet $P2Y_{12}$ receptor which prevents activation of the GPIIb/IIIa complex and platelet aggregation.

Dosage Form
- Oral (tablet)

Common Use
- Reduction of thrombotic events in patients with acute coronary syndrome or a history of MI

Quick Facts
- Black Box Warnings – Can cause significant and sometimes fatal bleeding and should not be used in patients with active pathological bleeding or history of intracranial hemorrhage. Do not start ticagrelor in patients undergoing urgent CABG surgery. Maintenance doses of aspirin above 100 mg reduce the effectiveness of ticagrelor and should be avoided.
- Avoid use with strong CYP3A4 inhibitors or inducers.
- Avoid concomitant use with simvastatin and lovastatin doses greater than 40 mg/day due to increased risk of myopathy.
- Avoid use in patients with severe hepatic impairment.
- Discontinue 5 days prior to elective surgery.
- Use ticagrelor with a daily maintenance dose of aspirin of 75 to 100 mg.
- Side effects: bleeding, dyspnea, dizziness, nausea

TIMOLOL (ophthalmic)

Brand Names
- Timoptic, Betimol, Istalol

Pharmacologic Class
- $Beta_1$/$beta_2$-blocker

Mechanism of Action
- Decreases intraocular pressure by reducing aqueous humor production and increasing uveoscleral outflow.

Dosage Forms
- Ophthalmic (solution, gel-forming solution)

Common Uses
- Treatment of open-angle glaucoma and ocular hypertension

Quick Facts
- Contraindications include active or history of bronchial asthma, 2nd or 3rd degree AV block, severe COPD, and sinus bradycardia.
- Systemic absorption is reduced when using nasolacrimal occlusion or closing the eyelids for 2 minutes after administration.
- Remove contact lenses before instilling medication and allow at least 15 minutes before reinserting.
- Administer other ophthalmic medications at least 10 minutes before using the gel-forming solution.
- Side effects: burning, stinging, or itching of eyes, blurred vision

TIOTROPIUM

Brand Names
- Spiriva, Spiriva Respimat

Pharmacologic Class
- Anticholinergic

Mechanism of Action
- Blocks the action of acetylcholine at parasympathetic sites in bronchial smooth muscle, causing bronchodilation.

Dosage Forms
- Inhalation (capsule, aerosol solution)

Common Uses
- Treatment of COPD and asthma (Respimat only)

Quick Facts
- Use with caution in patients with narrow-angle glaucoma, BPH, or bladder neck obstruction.
- When using the Spiriva HandiHaler, inhalation must be slow and sufficient to hear or feel the capsule vibrate. The capsules should not be opened before inserting in the HandiHaler device. Capsules must be stored in sealed blister packs. Clean the HandiHaler device with warm water at least once per month.
- Avoid getting aerosol spray or powder from capsules in eyes as this may cause eye pain, temporary blurring of vision, visual halos, mydriasis, or new onset or worsening of narrow-angle glaucoma.
- Side effects: dry mouth, pharyngitis, sinusitis, headache

TIZANIDINE

Brand Name
- Zanaflex

Pharmacologic Class
- Skeletal muscle relaxant

Mechanism of Action
- Agonist at alpha$_2$-adrenergic receptors and is thought to reduce spasticity by increasing presynaptic inhibition of motor neurons.

Dosage Forms
- Oral (tablet, capsule)

Common Use
- Treatment of spasticity

Quick Facts
- Tablets and capsules are bioequivalent under fasted conditions, but not under fed conditions. When taken with food, plasma concentrations of the tablet form are increased and the plasma concentrations of the capsule form are decreased.
- Monitor liver function during the first 6 months of treatment (baseline, 1, 3, and 6 months) and periodically thereafter.
- Use with caution when taken concurrently with other CNS depressants.
- Avoid abrupt discontinuation of medication. Rebound hypertension and tachycardia may occur.
- Avoid alcohol use.
- Side effects: drowsiness, dizziness, hypotension, dry mouth

TOLTERODINE

Brand Name
- Detrol

Pharmacologic Class
- Anticholinergic

Mechanism of Action
- Inhibits the muscarinic action of acetylcholine on smooth muscle, which causes bladder smooth muscle relaxation.

Dosage Forms
- Oral (tablet, capsule)

Common Use
- Treatment of overactive bladder

Quick Facts
- Contraindicated in patients with uncontrolled narrow-angle glaucoma, urinary retention, or gastric retention.
- Reduce dosage in renal impairment (CrCl < 30 mL/min).
- May be associated with QT prolongation.
- Increased drowsiness may occur with concomitant alcohol use.
- Side effects: dry mouth, headache, dizziness, constipation

TOPIRAMATE

Brand Names
- Topamax, Qudexy XR, Trokendi XR

Pharmacologic Class
- Anticonvulsant

Mechanism of Action
- Exact mechanism is unknown. Activity may be due to blocking voltage-dependent sodium channels, enhancing GABA-A activity, antagonizing AMPA/kainate glutamate receptors, and inhibiting carbonic anhydrase.

Dosage Forms
- Oral (tablet, capsule)

Common Uses
- Treatment of epilepsy (partial seizure, tonic-clonic seizure, Lennox-Gastaut syndrome); migraine prophylaxis

Quick Facts
- Medication may cause metabolic acidosis. Monitor serum bicarbonate at baseline and periodically during therapy.
- Decreased sweating and hyperthermia may occur, especially in pediatric patients.
- Taking during pregnancy increases the risk of oral cleft birth defects.
- Stay well hydrated during therapy to reduce the risk of kidney stone formation.
- Side effects: weight loss, abnormal vision, memory or concentration difficulties, fatigue

TORSEMIDE

Brand Name
- Demadex

Pharmacologic Class
- Loop diuretic

Mechanism of Action
- Inhibits sodium and chloride reabsorption in the proximal and distal tubules, as well as in the ascending loop of Henle.

Dosage Form
- Oral (tablet)

Common Uses
- Treatment of edema associated with heart failure, cirrhosis of the liver or renal disease, acute pulmonary edema, and hypertension

Quick Facts
- Contraindicated in patients with anuria.
- Medication can cause electrolyte imbalances including hypokalemia, hyponatremia, hypocalcemia, hypomagnesemia, and hypochloremic alkalosis. Monitor periodically.
- Tinnitus and hearing loss, usually reversible, has been reported. Higher than recommended doses, severe renal impairment, and hypoproteinemia may increase the risk.
- Administer in the morning due to increased diuresis.
- Use with caution in combination with NSAIDs due to the risk of acute renal failure.
- Side effects: hyperuricemia, hyperglycemia, headache, rash

TRAMADOL

Brand Names
- Ultram, ConZip

Pharmacologic Class
- Opioid analgesic

Mechanism of Action
- Binds to the mu opioid receptor, which reduces neuronal cell excitability and transmission of nociceptive impulses. Also inhibits the reuptake of norepinephrine and serotonin, which activate descending pain inhibitory pathways.

Dosage Forms
- Oral (tablet, capsule)

Common Use
- Treatment of moderate to severe pain

Quick Facts
- DEA Schedule IV
- Black Box Warnings – Serious, life-threatening, or fatal respiratory depression may occur. Concomitant use with benzodiazepines increases risk of sedation, respiratory depression, coma, or death. Concomitant use or discontinuation of CYP3A4 inducers, 3A4 inhibitors, or 2D6 inhibitors with tramadol requires careful consideration of the effects on tramadol and its active metabolite. Prolonged use of tramadol during pregnancy can result in neonatal opioid withdrawal syndrome. Contraindicated in children younger than 12 years of age and in children younger than 18 years of age following tonsillectomy and/or adenoidectomy.
- Seizures have been reported even when taken within the recommended dosage range. Risk is increased with doses exceeding the recommended range or with concomitant use with medications that decrease the seizure threshold, including SSRIs, TCAs, MAOIs, etc.
- Serotonin syndrome may occur, particularly with concomitant use of serotonergic medications.
- Side effects: pruritus, constipation, sweating, somnolence

TRAMADOL-ACETAMINOPHEN

Brand Name
- Ultracet

Pharmacologic Class
- Opioid analgesic combination

Mechanism of Action
- Tramadol binds to the mu opioid receptor, which reduces neuronal cell excitability and transmission of nociceptive impulses. It also inhibits the reuptake of norepinephrine and serotonin, which activate descending pain inhibitory pathways. Acetaminophen inhibits prostaglandin synthesis in the CNS and blocks pain impulse generation peripherally.

Dosage Form
- Oral (tablet)

Common Uses
- Treatment of moderate to severe pain

Quick Facts
- DEA Schedule IV
- Black Box Warnings – Serious, life-threatening, or fatal respiratory depression may occur. Concomitant use with benzodiazepines increases risk of sedation, respiratory depression, coma, or death. Concomitant use or discontinuation of CYP3A4 inducers, 3A4 inhibitors, or 2D6 inhibitors with tramadol requires careful consideration of the effects on tramadol and its active metabolite. Prolonged use of tramadol during pregnancy can result in neonatal opioid withdrawal syndrome. Contraindicated in children younger than 12 years of age and in children younger than 18 years of age following tonsillectomy and/or adenoidectomy.
- Tramadol can increase seizure risk and serotonin syndrome risk. Acetaminophen has been associated with cases of acute liver failure.
- Patients should not exceed more than 4 grams of acetaminophen in a 24-hour period.
- Side effects: pruritis, constipation, sweating, somnolence

TRAVOPROST

Brand Name
- Travatan Z

Pharmacologic Class
- Prostaglandin analog

Mechanism of Action
- Decreases intraocular pressure by increasing the outflow of aqueous humor through the trabecular meshwork and uveoscleral pathway.

Dosage Form
- Ophthalmic (solution)

Common Uses
- Treatment of open-angle glaucoma and ocular hypertension

Quick Facts
- Remove contact lenses before instilling medication and allow at least 15 minutes before reinserting.
- Wait at least 5 minutes before administering other ophthalmic products.
- Side effects: pigment changes to eyelids and eyelashes, increased brown pigmentation of the iris, growth of eyelashes, conjunctival hyperemia, ocular pruritis

TRAZODONE

Brand Names
- Desyrel, Oleptro

Pharmacologic Class
- SARI (Serotonin antagonist and reuptake inhibitor)

Mechanism of Action
- Inhibits the neuronal reuptake of serotonin and acts as an antagonist at 5-HT$_{2A/2C}$ serotonin receptors. Also blocks histamine and alpha$_1$-adrenergic receptors.

Dosage Form
- Oral (tablet)

Common Uses
- Treatment of insomnia and depression

Quick Facts
- Black Box Warning – Increased risk of suicidal thoughts and behavior in children, adolescents, and young adults.
- Use is contraindicated during or within 14 days of MAOI administration.
- May cause QT prolongation.
- Grapefruit juice and CYP3A4 inhibitors can increase levels of trazodone.
- Immediate-release tablets should be taken after a meal or light snack. Extended-release tablets should be taken on an empty stomach.
- Side effects: drowsiness, orthostatic hypotension, syncope, priapism

TRIAMCINOLONE (topical)

Brand Name
- Kenalog

Pharmacologic Class
- Corticosteroid

Mechanism of Action
- Has anti-inflammatory, antipruritic, and vasoconstrictive properties. The anti-inflammatory effect is believed to be due to stimulation of phospholipase A_2 inhibitory proteins. These proteins subsequently block the release of arachidonic acid, which is a precursor to leukotrienes and prostaglandins.

Dosage Forms
- Topical (cream, ointment, spray, lotion), dental paste

Common Uses
- Treatment of inflammatory and pruritic manifestations of corticosteroid-responsive dermatoses; dental paste is used for the treatment of oral inflammatory and ulcerative lesions

Quick Facts
- Topical steroid overuse can cause thinning of the skin and striae.
- Do not use with bandages, wraps, or other occlusive dressings unless directed by prescriber.
- Apply sparingly and wash hands after application.
- To use the dental paste, press a small dab onto the mouth ulcer but do not rub in. The dab will form a thin film that should be left in place for several hours. The dental paste is usually applied at bedtime and/or after meals.
- Side effects: pruritis, burning sensation, hypothalamic-pituitary-adrenal axis suppression

TRIAMTERENE-HYDROCHLOROTHIAZIDE

Brand Names
- Dyazide, Maxzide

Pharmacologic Class
- Combination thiazide and potassium-sparing diuretic

Mechanism of Action
- Triamterene inhibits the reabsorption of sodium in the renal distal convoluted tubule in exchange for potassium. Hydrochlorothiazide inhibits sodium and chloride reabsorption in the renal distal convoluted tubule.

Dosage Forms
- Oral (tablet, capsule)

Common Uses
- Treatment of edema and hypertension

Quick Facts
- Black Box Warning – Hyperkalemia can occur with triamterene. Risk is increased in patients with renal impairment, diabetes, and the elderly or severely ill. Monitor potassium levels at frequent intervals.
- Contraindications include anuria, acute or chronic renal insufficiency, or significant renal impairment and hyperkalemia.
- Administer in the morning because of increased diuresis.
- Patients should avoid potassium supplements and foods containing high levels of potassium, including salt substitutes.
- Drink plenty of fluids when using oral form to prevent renal toxicity.
- Side effects: hyperuricemia, hyperglycemia, rash, photosensitivity

VALACYCLOVIR

Brand Name
- Valtrex

Pharmacologic Class
- Antiviral

Mechanism of Action
- Valacyclovir is a prodrug and is converted to acyclovir by intestinal and hepatic metabolism. Acyclovir is converted to the active triphosphate form, which interferes with viral DNA polymerase and inhibits viral DNA replication.

Dosage Form
- Oral (tablet)

Common Uses
- Treatment of genital herpes, herpes zoster (shingles), herpes labialis (cold sores), and varicella zoster (chickenpox)

Quick Facts
- Treatment with valacyclovir should be initiated at the earliest sign of a cold sore, genital herpes, or chickenpox, and as soon as possible after a diagnosis of herpes zoster.
- Drink plenty of fluids during therapy to prevent renal toxicity. Take with food if GI upset occurs.
- CNS reactions such as agitation, hallucinations, confusion, and encephalopathy have been reported. Use with caution in elderly patients and reduce dosage in patients with renal impairment.
- Side effects: headache, nausea, abdominal pain

VALSARTAN

Brand Name
- Diovan

Pharmacologic Class
- ARB

Mechanism of Action
- Blocks the binding of angiotensin II to the angiotensin II type-1 receptor on vascular smooth muscle, which prevents vasoconstriction and the secretion of aldosterone.

Dosage Form
- Oral (tablet)

Common Uses
- Treatment of hypertension and heart failure (NYHA Class II-IV); reduction of cardiovascular mortality in patients with left ventricular dysfunction or failure post-MI

Quick Facts
- Black Box Warning – Discontinue use as soon as possible if pregnancy is detected.
- Contraindicated with concomitant use with aliskiren in diabetic patients.
- NSAIDs may reduce antihypertensive effect and increase the risk of renal dysfunction.
- Patients should avoid potassium supplements or salt substitutes containing potassium without first consulting healthcare provider.
- Side effects: dizziness, headache, fatigue, increased blood urea nitrogen

VALSARTAN-HYDROCHLOROTHIAZIDE

Brand Name
- Diovan HCT

Pharmacologic Class
- Combination ARB and thiazide diuretic

Mechanism of Action
- Valsartan blocks the binding of angiotensin II to the angiotensin II type-1 receptor on vascular smooth muscle, which prevents vasoconstriction and the secretion of aldosterone. Hydrochlorothiazide inhibits sodium and chloride reabsorption in the renal distal convoluted tubule.

Dosage Form
- Oral (tablet)

Common Use
- Treatment of hypertension

Quick Facts
- Black Box Warning – Discontinue use as soon as possible if pregnancy is detected.
- Contraindicated in patients with anuria, concomitant use with aliskiren in diabetic patients, and hypersensitivity to sulfonamides.
- Administer in the morning because of increased diuresis.
- Patients should avoid potassium supplements or salt substitutes containing potassium without first consulting healthcare provider.
- Side effects: dizziness, pharyngitis, increased blood urea nitrogen, fatigue

VARDENAFIL

Brand Names
- Levitra, Staxyn

Pharmacologic Class
- PDE-5 inhibitor

Mechanism of Action
- Inhibits phosphodiesterase-5, which increases levels of cyclic guanosine monophosphate (cGMP) within vascular smooth muscle cells, causing relaxation and vasodilation.

Dosage Forms
- Oral (tablet, orally disintegrating tablet)

Common Use
- Treatment of erectile dysfunction

Quick Facts
- Concomitant use with organic nitrates is contraindicated due to the risk of hypotension.
- Taking medication with a high fat meal slows absorption.
- Take approximately 1 hour before sexual activity and with at least 24 hours between doses.
- Patients should be counseled to immediately report priapism, vision loss in one or both eyes, and sudden decrease or loss of hearing.
- Side effects: flushing, headache, dizziness, dyspepsia, rhinitis

VARENICLINE

Brand Name
- Chantix

Pharmacologic Class
- Partial nicotine agonist

Mechanism of Action
- Binds to alpha$_4$beta$_2$ neuronal nicotinic receptors where it produces agonist activity while simultaneously preventing nicotine binding to these receptors. Also stimulates dopamine activity to a small degree, resulting in decreased craving and withdrawal symptoms.

Dosage Form
- Oral (tablet)

Common Use
- Aid to smoking cessation treatment

Quick Facts
- Serious neuropsychiatric symptoms may occur, including changes in behavior, agitation, depression, and suicidal ideation. Use with caution in patients with underlying psychiatric disorders.
- Patients should report symptoms of angina, MI, stroke, and skin rash with mucosal lesions.
- Begin therapy 1 week prior to quit date chosen by patient. Alternatively, patient may begin therapy and then set a quit date between days 8 and 35 of treatment.
- Take after meals and with a full glass of water.
- Reduce dosage in renal impairment (CrCl < 30 mL/min).
- Side effects: nausea, abnormal dreams, constipation, insomnia, headache

VENLAFAXINE

Brand Name
- Effexor

Pharmacologic Class
- SNRI

Mechanism of Action
- Increases the synaptic concentration of serotonin and norepinephrine in the CNS by inhibiting their reuptake at presynaptic nerve terminals. Also weakly inhibits the reuptake of dopamine.

Dosage Forms
- Oral (tablet, capsule)

Common Uses
- Treatment of depression, generalized anxiety disorder, panic disorder, and social anxiety disorder

Quick Facts
- Black Box Warning – Increased risk of suicidal thoughts and behavior, especially in children, adolescents, and young adults.
- Do not abruptly discontinue medication.
- Symptomatic improvement may take several weeks.
- Use is contraindicated during or within 14 days of MAOI administration, and allow 7 days after stopping venlafaxine before starting an MAOI.
- Monitor blood pressure regularly.
- Side effects: nausea, dry mouth, constipation, hypertension, sweating, sexual dysfunction in men

VERAPAMIL

Brand Names
- Calan, Verelan

Pharmacologic Class
- Calcium channel blocker

Mechanism of Action
- Non-dihydropyridine CCB that blocks the transmembrane influx of calcium ions into vascular smooth muscle and cardiac muscle which results in increased peripheral arterial vasodilation and decreased peripheral vascular resistance. Also is a negative inotrope (decreased force) and negative chronotrope (decreased rate).

Dosage Forms
- Oral (tablet, capsule), intravenous (solution)

Common Uses
- Treatment of hypertension, paroxysmal supraventricular tachycardia, atrial fibrillation, and angina (chronic stable, unstable, and variant)

Quick Facts
- Contraindications include 2nd or 3rd degree AV block without a functioning pacemaker, hypotension (SBP < 90 mmHg), and severe left ventricular dysfunction.
- Medication is both a substrate and inhibitor CYP3A4.
- Do not abruptly discontinue medication.
- Side effects: peripheral edema, constipation, headache, dizziness

VILAZODONE

Brand Name
- Viibryd

Pharmacologic Class
- SSRI/5-HT$_{1A}$ receptor partial agonist

Mechanism of Action
- Inhibits the reuptake of serotonin in presynaptic neurons of the CNS. Also a partial agonist of 5-HT$_{1A}$ receptors, but the effect in depression is unknown.

Dosage Form
- Oral (tablet)

Common Use
- Treatment of depression

Quick Facts
- Black Box Warning – Increased risk of suicidal thoughts and behavior in children, adolescents, and young adults.
- May increase the risk of bleeding events. Concomitant use of aspirin, NSAIDs, warfarin, and other anticoagulants can increase risk.
- Use is contraindicated during or within 14 days of MAOI administration, and allow 14 days after stopping vilazodone before starting an MAOI.
- Administer with food.
- Do not abruptly discontinue medication.
- Patients should report symptoms of hyponatremia, including headache, confusion, and weakness.
- Side effects: diarrhea, nausea, vomiting, insomnia

WARFARIN

Brand Names
- Coumadin, Jantoven

Pharmacologic Class
- Anticoagulant

Mechanism of Action
- Blocks the function of the vitamin K epoxide reductase complex, which inhibits the synthesis of vitamin-K dependent clotting factors (II, VII, IX, and X) and proteins C and S.

Dosage Form
- Oral (tablet)

Common Uses
- Prophylaxis and treatment of venous thrombosis, arising pulmonary embolisms, and thromboembolic complications from atrial fibrillation or cardiac valve replacement; used to reduce the risk of death, recurrent MI, and thromboembolic events (e.g., stroke, systemic embolization) after MI

Quick Facts
- Black Box Warning – Warfarin can cause major or fatal bleeding. All treated patients should have regular INR monitoring. Drugs, dietary changes, and other factors affect INR levels. Instruct patients about prevention measures to minimize risk of bleeding and to report signs and symptoms of bleeding.
- Inhibitors and inducers of CYP2C9, 1A2, or 3A4 may affect warfarin levels.
- Patients should contact prescriber immediately if they have symptoms of purple toe syndrome or warfarin-induced skin necrosis.
- Dietary vitamin K must be consistent.
- Side effects: nausea, abdominal pain, rash, chills

ZIPRASIDONE

Brand Name
- Geodon

Pharmacologic Class
- Antipsychotic

Mechanism of Action
- Blocks dopamine D_2 and serotonin 5-HT_{2A} receptors. Also blocks histamine H_1 and alpha$_1$-adrenergic receptors.

Dosage Forms
- Oral (capsule), intramuscular (powder for solution)

Common Uses
- Treatment of bipolar disorder and schizophrenia

Quick Facts
- Black Box Warning – Elderly patients with dementia-related psychosis treated with antipsychotics are at an increased risk of death compared to placebo. Most deaths appeared to be either cardiovascular (e.g., heart failure, sudden death) or infectious (e.g., pneumonia) in nature.
- Can prolong the QT interval.
- Patients should be counseled to report signs of extrapyramidal symptoms, tardive dyskinesia (restlessness, tremor, stiffness, etc.) or neuroleptic malignant syndrome (sweating, fever, muscle rigidity, etc.).
- Monitor for hyperglycemia, dyslipidemia, and weight gain.
- Administer oral capsules with food to increase absorption.
- Side effects: somnolence, dizziness, nausea, rash

ZOLPIDEM

Brand Names
- Ambien, Edluar, Intermezzo

Pharmacologic Class
- Hypnotic

Mechanism of Action
- Increases the activity of GABA by selective agonism at the benzodiazepine-1 receptor.

Dosage Forms
- Oral (tablet, sublingual tablet, spray)

Common Use
- Treatment of insomnia

Quick Facts
- DEA Schedule IV
- Black Box Warning – Complex sleep behaviors including sleep-walking, sleep-driving, and engaging in other activities while not fully awake may occur. Discontinue medication immediately if a patient experiences a complex sleep behavior. Use is contraindicated in patients who have experienced these events.
- Administer medication immediately before bedtime. Do not take with or immediately following a meal, as it may delay onset.
- Avoid alcohol and other CNS depressants.
- Side effects in short-term trials: drowsiness, dizziness
- Side effects in long-term trials: dizziness, drugged feelings, lethargy

INDEX

Made in the USA
Coppell, TX
21 January 2022